YOGA

on

WAR

and

PEACE

D1304568

YOGA

— on —

WAR

— and —

PEACE

Pandit Rajmani Tigunait Ph.D.

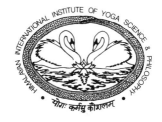

**Published by
The Himalayan International Institute
of Yoga Science and Philosophy of the U.S.A.
Honesdale, Pennsylvania**

© 1991 by The Himalayan International Institute
of Yoga Science and Philosophy of the U.S.A.
RR 1, Box 400 / Honesdale, Pennsylvania 18431

First Printing 1991

All rights reserved. Reproduction of this book in any manner, in whole or in part, in English or in any other language, is prohibited without the written permission of the publisher. Printed in the United States of America.

The paper used in this publication meets the minimum requirements of American National Standard for Information Science—Permanence of Paper for Printed Library Materials, ANSI Z39.48-1984.

Tigunait, Rajmani, 1953–
        Yoga on war and peace / Rajmani Tigunait.
            p. cm.
        ISBN 0-89389-125-8
        1. War—Religious aspects. 2. Peace—Religious aspects. 3. Yoga.
    I. Title.
    BL65.W23T54 1991
    294.5'17873—dc20   91-14248
                                                            CIP

Dedication

This book is dedicated to
The human race—
Civilians and soldiers,
Foes and friends,
Women and men,
Old and young.
May it find and
Touch all hearts
Seeking peace, and the
End of wars.

Contents

Invocation

May the whole world be happy.
May our bodies and minds be free of sickness.
May the world attain only that which is auspicious.
May no one partake of the pain of violence.

Peace, Peace, Peace.

Message

I came not to judge the world but to save the world.

The New Testament
John 12:47

The Lord of Life and
The Lord of the Universe
Lives enshrined in
You and me
Her and him.
Let Him shine
Within and without.
Dismantle not, oh mankind,
The living shrine
This beautiful temple
From which He shines. . . .

Sages from the Past

Forward

— True nonresistance is the one true resistance to evil. It kills and finally destroys the evil sentiment.

Leo Tolstoy

— My optimism rests on my belief in the infinite possibilities of the individual to develop nonviolence. The more you develop it in your own being, the more it overwhelms your surroundings and by and by might oversweep the world.

M.K. Gandhi

War is an eternal problem. The question of how a person of conscience responds to war or violence has engaged the thoughts and emotions of many of the wisest people throughout all eras and across a variety of cultures. Is there such a thing as a just war? On what basis does a man or woman decide to participate in taking the lives of others? How do we end war? Is it even possible to do so? Since the atomic weapons used in World War II shocked the world with their destructive power, great social, political, and spiritual attention has been devoted to the goal of peace. Active, spiritually minded individuals have dedicated themselves to addressing the problems of violence and war in a number of arenas—among them, the civil rights movement, the peace movement of the Vietnam war era, movements to end ecological violence, and the programs for famine relief around the world. All are evidence of a growing sense of kinship and involvement with a larger social community.

And yet wars go on and violence continues to erupt throughout the world—violence between countries and within communities; violence between diverse groups, and within families. In the face of each new conflict we ask ourselves how we will ever stem this tide of hatred, violence, and war.

In this beautiful and timely book, Pandit Rajmani Tigunait considers the implications of yoga and spiritual teachings for the problem of war and peace. What is even more important, he offers the thoughtful reader a program of personal commitment to real peace.

Just as many are committed to involvement in activities that seek to eliminate the seeds of war and hatred in the external social and political world, so also is there a need to extract the internal seeds of war by eliminating those aspects within the human mind and heart that block our progress toward achieving peace. This is a program of inner transformation and evolution for those who are sincerely committed to real peace.

This quiet and inspiring book shares practices and contemplations that will help those working for peace to cultivate peace within while eliminating all seeds of violence. Those who dedicate themselves to this task will find that this process of inner self-transformation is a complement to the external process of engendering political and social change. It is in this internal process of uprooting the causes of war that we will meet our greatest challenge.

Kay Gendron, Ph.D.

Acknowledgements

I express my gratitude to my Master, who chooses me to deliver his message of peace and nonviolence. Paths and maps were already prepared by the sages. I simply re-presented them here in modern terms with the help of my colleagues and all the fellow seekers who lent their energy to this project, directly and indirectly.

One

Even flowers in wild and lonely places, which bloom and drop their petals back to dust, have purpose, although it be beyond your ken. The Creator knows; that is enough.

The Pre-War Crisis

Why Do We Fight?

N o one likes war, yet war is perennial. Everyone knows the value of peace, yet we are restless without some unrest. Just as we are addicted to a variety of destructive habits at the individual level, at the collective level we are addicted to wars, riots, political upheavals, and religious crusades. Yet, each time we fight, we pay a heavy price. The apparent winners often lose more than those who suffer defeat on the battlefield.

Before a war breaks out, each side loudly proclaims its own righteousness and the opponent's wickedness. The populace becomes absorbed in vilifying the "enemy." Emotions are inflamed, war fever takes over, and little energy remains for finding a nonviolent solution. Before the war begins, both parties claim that they are messengers of peace; sometimes the leaders even claim to be prophets

or saviors. If one side presents a peaceful option for set-
tling the dispute and this proposal is rejected, then the
issue becomes one of national pride or political vanity and
the prime goal—peace itself—is forgotten.

Anyone with common sense knows this is true—we
say we want peace, yet we wage war. By the time a war
has run its appalling course, everyone is sickened by the
slaughter, the torn and blackened landscape, the ruined
cities, and the shattered lives. People from both sides—
winners and losers, civilians and soldiers, leaders and
citizens—vow never to go to war again. But alas, human
memory is short. Forgetting the lessons of the past, and
failing to understand the reasons that we fight, we soon
find ourselves embroiled again.

Several millennia ago, the sages of the yoga tradition
pondered these matters and concluded that the causes of
such man-made catastrophes are more subtle than we
usually think. In the past, gold, gems, land, religious beliefs, and women were the overt reasons for war. In modern times, women are no longer given as an excuse, but the
other elements remain unchanged.

According to yoga, stopping the cycle of war requires
delving into the subtle causes underlying the surface mo-
tives of material gain and religious differences. These
subtle causes are selfishness, ego, greed, ethnocentrism,
and inferiority complexes. Due to these, we fail to do what
we know is right and persist in doing what we know is
wrong. In the scriptures, this phenomenon is called killing

the conscience. The great scriptures of yoga—*The Bhagavad Gita, The Yoga Sutra,* and *The Upanishads*—clearly describe how the subtle causes of external war emanate from the internal world. The real causes of war lie rooted in the individual's unwillingness to listen to the voice of the heart, the inner conscience.

Looking into Subtle Causes

Wars are not the fault of armies or governments. Soldiers are not alien beings, but our relatives and neighbors. Their thoughts and feelings are like ours. Fighting is their job, but if given a choice, they will avoid violence the same as a civilian. The duty of a soldier is to protect the other members of society from harm, and the government officials who order them to fight are also doing their duty, which is to guide, govern, and preserve the social order. Violence does not originate with soldiers or the governments that employ them. Rather, it originates with the most basic unit of society—the individual.

The problem begins even before birth. Each baby is born into a religious structure; a well-defined group awareness; a certain economic class; a particular race, caste, color, faith, and creed; and a set of superstitions and dogmas. The moment a child enters the world, the parents begin to impart this sense of divisiveness and to impose it on their offspring. Thus, we enter the world already entangled in a web of labels and identities, which we gradually come to believe and to mistake for ourselves. We grow into adulthood wedded to these superficial identities, a sense of "I am" one trait or another.

Our entire value system is shaped by the elements we have absorbed from our upbringing. Differences in value systems arise from differing backgrounds, and because we identify with our values, those with different values become a threat to our sense of "I-am-ness." Even the higher values of love and compassion become confined to those who share our values. That is why we teach and preach the values of love and compassion while judging and hating those who do not belong to our own little group.

We believe that we value universal brotherhood and sisterhood, but our concept of brotherhood and sisterhood is quite limited. If a wife and husband who believe in two different faiths quarrel over which religious values to teach their children, and finally settle the matter by divorcing and splitting the children, what can you expect of two different cultures? Have you ever heard of a Moslem adopting a child from Christian parents and raising that child as a Christian? That would be a miracle, and the person raising such a child would be a great soul.

According to yoga, there is a collective awareness just as there is an individual awareness. A family is made of its members. A community consists of several families, a society of several communities, and a nation of several societies. Just as children in the family fight over toys, families and communities also quarrel with each other. A community consisting of several families stands on a common ground of shared values. On the basis of these values, it distinguishes itself from other communities. During the years the ego is developing, every child thinks that he or she is better than other children. The same tendency can be observed with communities. As human beings and communities mature, they leave behind trivial matters and become adult. However, this is possible only if the most important factor—ego—is transformed, expanded, refined, and polished. Ego, "I-am-ness," is the greatest barrier in the transformation and development of an individual at a personal level and, therefore, of society at the collective level.

This is where yoga steps in. According to yoga, the primary task of the individual is to overcome the trivial sense of "I-am-ness," or *asmita*. As long as we are stuck with the idea of "I am good," "I am bad," "I am Christian," "I am Moslem," "I am American," "I am Indian," "I am superior," "I am inferior," "I am poor," "I am rich," we can help neither ourselves nor others. Instead we remain embroiled in the exhausting chore of feeding the ego we have mistaken for ourselves, while holding the mask we have assumed firmly in place.

In order to satisfy the ego momentarily, we judge others and take delight in interfering with their lives under the illusion that we are uniquely qualified to set others straight. Because we are unhappy with ourselves, we attempt to force others to surrender to us, hoping that their submission will convince us of our worth, thereby increasing our happiness. However, other people are caught in the same behavior, even those whom we regard as inferior.

Every community and society consists of individuals who are absorbed in this deception, and collectively such individuals create a grander, collective ego. There are many such collectives—ethnic groups, nations, sects, and factions of every persuasion. It is because of this collective ego that communities form nations and nations form alliances. It is because of this ego that East and West, First World and Third World emerge.

The Yoga Sutra, the most prominent yoga text, says that attachment and aversion evolve directly from this sense of "I-am-ness." No matter how terrible our self-image, it is extremely difficult to shed that image and replace it with a healthier one because of the powerful attachment to that original sense of "I am." Because of this attachment, we are reluctant to examine this sense of "I am" to discover whether it is real or not. Due to this attachment, we delight in imposing the superficial grandeur of our "I-am-ness" on others. If others resist, we feel angry. When others attempt to impose their egos on us or on others, we consider them to be competitors. When we notice that another's self-image consists of healthier and more attractive elements than our own, we become envious. Thus anger, animosity, and jealousy are born.

If the global community consists mostly of individuals

who have not worked with their egos, there will be no end to war in the outside world. War is the result of the intrinsic vanity of both the individual and the collective ego of mankind. Ego suffers from poverty, vanity, and emptiness, and it attempts to mask this sense of void by acquiring worldly objects, name, fame, dignity, and status. Lacking internal fulfillment, it tries to compensate with objects that do not belong to it in the first place. History is replete with examples of land, wealth, and property being used to compensate for inner emptiness and to satisfy the ego's vanity. Under the influence of vanity, the ego claims ownership of objects which were not earned through rightful means, and comes up against another ego making the same claims. Thus, the interests of two individual or collective egos clash, and peace and harmony are destroyed.

According to the yoga scriptures, ego has an enormous appetite. The name of that appetite is desire. A human being has insatiable desires, and in the process of fulfilling them, forgets that others are also suffering from the same uncontrollable appetites. The ego forgets that it is impossible to possess the whole world. It forgets that others have the same urges and that therefore, its impulses will clash with those of others and will lead to chaos.

How much land does a king, a shah, or an emperor need? How much wealth does it take to satisfy one who craves wealth? What is the highest status and the most potent symbol of power that a power-hungry person can achieve? There is no limit to such urges. And unless we learn how to erect a stop sign, we cannot avoid a crash. Unless we come to understand the self-defeating nature of our possessiveness, we cannot stop making war. By the time one war has ended, people will already be gathering their forces for another war, one after another. And all these good guys and bad guys will keep emerging because they are reflections of ourselves.

It is entirely useless to try to figure out who is right and who is wrong, who is good and who is bad. The pressing task is to create a state of well-being, a state of individual and social health, of peace and concord—a state where all forces, all tendencies, all elements can come into harmony and human beings can live together peacefully.

Possessiveness is a sickness. The accumulation of excessive material objects is debilitating. This is true at both individual and collective levels. A society that is deprived of higher spiritual values substitutes a purely materialistic worldview and, as a result, loses the ability to discriminate between real needs and uncontrolled desires. Such a society fails to share the gifts of nature and the gifts of God with the rest of humanity. History is laden with examples of this malaise.

This is not to say that yoga encourages poverty or discourages worldly prosperity. Yoga simply says, "Remember, this whole world with all its objects has evolved from God and still exists in God. Every single object, every single aspect of this world is pervaded by God. Things of the world are given to you as gifts. Learn to enjoy them without becoming attached to them. While enjoying the objects of the world, make sure that you do not covet others' wealth." (*Isha Upanishad*, verse I.)

Once we understand that every entity, including ourselves, and every worldly object has evolved from that single Truth and that everything in this world is pervaded by that one Truth, we will not fight over objects that ultimately belong to that Truth and not to us. The knowledge that we are privileged to have all these worldly resources at our disposal and yet we are not the owners will protect us from disputes and disagreements.

The problem is that our self-centered ego does not allow us to adopt a perspective from which such a conclusion can be derived. Thus, we are left with the problem of how to manage our selfishness, ego, greed, and desires. These subtle problems can be solved neither through political negotiations nor with sermons. The only way to overcome these subtle causes of our external catastrophes lies in applying spiritual tools and committing ourselves to the disciplines that lead us to self-transformation.

A pragmatic politician may argue "Well, this is all very noble and philosophically soothing, but how does it apply to the emergencies of the moment?"

A yogi would respond: "General awareness is more powerful than the decisions of an individual or a handful of people. The enlightened multitude can stop the injustice brought about by a handful of people. Didn't the great soul, Mahatma Gandhi, lead a peaceful war in South

Africa and India and finally win, not simply the war, but the hearts of those who staunchly opposed him? Such a thing can be done. It requires courage, tolerance, forbearance, endurance, and a total commitment to practice the philosophy one professes, but it *is* possible. The great scripture, *The Bhagavad Gita*, says, 'Peace is priceless. Attain peace at any cost.'"

The pragmatist will counter that this is all very well but it does not solve the immediate problem, and that furthermore, it takes a long time to create a new, nonviolent collective awareness. In responding to such arguments, we must remember that here we are talking, not about the current problem, but rather about all the war situations still to come. Neither history nor the human race is so short-lived. Even if it takes twenty years, fifty years, or a hundred years to create the collective awareness of nonviolence, it will still be a noble achievement and we should set about it now.

The Consequences of Hatred and Revenge

We must shed the delusion that it is possible to attain peace through unpeaceful means. Here is the reason why: both parties in a war strongly believe that they are fighting for a just end. Both parties are supported by people who believe in similar goals. When a war is fought, lives are lost and natural and man-made resources are destroyed. It is true that in the modern world many nations come forward after a war with aid and funds for the damaged countries, but no amount of aid will heal the emotional injuries or quell the hatred in the hearts of the survivors.

The injury and oppression people suffered during World War II still lingers, even after the lapse of almost half a century. Hatred for the oppressors persists, engendering unrest and violence in countries like the Soviet Union and in European and Middle Eastern nations. After any war, people nourish their vengeful thoughts and their hatred. Vengeance and hatred are like molten rock seething underground. This magma builds up during the so-called "peace period." Sooner or later, it is bound to explode.

The post-war period is the time when the magma of revenge and hatred begins to form. War is simply the explosion. The magma breaks through the weakest spot, turning that region into a volcano. There are many weak spots in our global society that are subject to periodic eruptions of revenge and hatred.

It is important to provide humanitarian aid when the volcano explodes and to ease the misery of those who are in its path. And it is vital to bring such an explosion to an end as skillfully as possible. However, the crucial task is to prevent the magma from accumulating again. This can only be done by eradicating the fear, greed, selfishness, and anger from which the magma of revenge and hatred arises. This requires adopting an approach that has the power to effect a dramatic transformation—a "spiritual" approach.

This qualitative transformation must begin with the individual. Because society consists of individuals, individual transformation will give rise to a transformed society. Whenever we ignore the need for individual transformation and emphasize social transformation instead, a political or religious movement usually results, and transformation gives way to social reform or a "movement" of some sort. Eventually the leaders become ensnared by ego and vanity, and the movement either collapses or its integrity is compromised.

A spiritual approach that emphasizes individual purification and transformation runs no risk of sacrificing the higher values. It is also more lasting than social transformation. Once the number of individuals who have transformed themselves reaches a critical mass, social transformation occurs automatically. Furthermore, individual transformation has an immediate effect on the lives of children, whereas a mass movement only affects adults. What we do for our children is critical because it lays the groundwork for individual and collective transformation of future generations.

Individual transformation has the further advantage of being easier for our families, societies, and nations to absorb. The higher virtues can be developed in a relaxed manner and society can be spared the shock of revolution. Revolutions, even in the best causes, always create unrest and usually involve bloodshed. Individual transformation avoids such cataclysms. It is for this reason that Buddha repeatedly proclaimed, "Light your own lamp and the lives of others will be illuminated effortlessly." None of us has the power to force others to rid themselves of darkness. The only power we have is to demonstrate how delightful it is to live in the light.

According to yoga philosophy, there is a definite method of attaining inner peace and illumination, and there is a definite method of letting this light shine forth. This method of self-transformation gently unfolds the virtues of nonviolence, love, and compassion. In order to be healthy, happy, and loving, we must create a bridge between our body and mind, mind and soul, inner and external worlds, and our worldly life and our spiritual life.

Real transformation requires that we close the chasm between our worldly life and our spiritual life. Only then can we hold dual citizenship in two worlds—the world outside and the world inside. For this reason, the ancient masters invented a method of transformation that simultaneously affects every aspect of life: body, breath, mind, soul, and interpersonal relationships. As the following pages will demonstrate, such methods involve paying attention to what we eat; how we eat, think, behave, and communicate with others; how we view this world; and how we maintain our status and position without threatening the status and position of others. This method is the practice of *ahimsa*—nonviolence.

Preparation for Transformation: Eight Practical Steps

As with many other powerful practices, the practice of nonviolence requires preparation. The basic requirement is the proper mental state—it is impossible to practice nonviolence with a disturbed mind. Contemplation is a proven means of calming and clearing the mind. There are eight steps of contemplative practice which, if followed, will engender a worldview and philosophy of life that will support the practice of nonviolence. These steps are right views, right resolve, right speech, right conduct, right livelihood, right effort, right mindfulness, and right meditation. What follows is a glimpse of the method of applying these principles and making them an integral part of your life.

Choose a specific time every day to practice these contemplative techniques. Make yourself available at that time, free yourself from worldly concerns, and attend to your own thoughts and feelings lovingly and respectfully. As thoughts flash in the mind, pay attention to them. As you contemplate these principles, try to feel what you think. This is a dialogue between the unawakened and wakened soul within you. You are both orator and audience, teacher and student, counselor and client. You are both subject and object. As the thoughts flow and emotions are evoked, let them form themselves as tears or smiles, let them manifest silently or verbally—let them stir your entire being. Let the deepest core of your heart be touched by these contemplative thoughts. Do not reserve any privacy. Let the spirit of Buddha or Christ, Krishna or Moses sink into you and expand your sense of "I-am-ness" beyond the realm of boundaries.

In the beginning, you might simply read through the words written here. Later, it will not be the words, but the content of the words that pervades your mind, uplifts your soul, and transforms your entire being. At that stage, no one can tell you how much time you should spend in contemplation. It becomes your wealth, and wherever your wealth is, there will your heart be also.

1. Right Thought

Sit comfortably in a tranquil environment, preferably with your head, neck, and trunk straight. Withdraw your mind from external sounds. Focus on yourself—your body, your breath, and your mind. For a moment think of those who are near and dear to you. Recall the circumstances of the life you are living. Select a particular area of your life and reflect on how permanent or transitory it is, how much pain or pleasure it involves. Now begin the dialogue with your mind:

Mind, what makes you miserable? Worldly objects? Friends or foes? Losses or gains? And

ultimately, mind, don't you realize that everything, including yourself, your beloved ones, and all the objects of the world are impermanent? In this short span of life, you get attached to things and to people; you create expectations that cannot be fulfilled by anyone. You forget that you have come to this plane to accomplish something and after accomplishing it, you will leave everything behind and move on. Mind, how ignorant you are that you mistake the impermanent for the permanent; that is why your expectations are so high. And, mind, if you don't change your attitude, you will end up with the same frustrations you have experienced many times in the past.

Objects of the world are neither painful nor pleasant. In their absolute sense, they are neither good nor bad. Conditioned to time and place, everything in the world, including our fellow beings, keeps changing its shape, behavior, and attitudes; and thus, from moment to moment, different characteristics of the same thing manifest differently. You expected that your car would always run smoothly— that was your mistake. So when it got a flat tire today, you upset yourself.

Mind, you must learn how to work hard and yet, take it lightly. You must learn how to love others selflessly, without any expectation. You will find delight only when you do what you are supposed to do without expecting others to do what they are supposed to do. If they fail to do what they are supposed to do, that is normal. Drop your habit of blaming and criticizing others. Listen to the sage who said: 'Tell me, how many people are there in the world who magnify a virtue the size of a mustard seed in a fellow being into the size of the Himalayas and thus adore and worship only the virtue?'

Mind, it is entirely up to you what you look for and therefore, what you find. Change your attitude. Look for good, you will find it. Seek contentment, you will find it. Search for happiness, you will find it. This world is filled with everything you want— good or bad, pleasant or unpleasant, right or wrong, pain or pleasure, friends or enemies. What you search for is entirely up to you.

In different sittings, you can change the tone of your contemplation. You can address yourself, your mind, or humanity. You can pick a particular principle, theme, or idea that flashes strongly in your mind. For example, you might pick inhumanity itself as a theme and reach a conclusion that will help you expand your worldview. Thus:

What has happened to you, mankind, that you suffer on account of not having enough but care nothing about destroying that which you already have? Such is human nature. Self-destructive tendencies walk side by side with uplifting, creative tendencies.

Mind, if you can stop the destructive forces, then stop them. If you cannot, then let them be. But in either case, don't pollute yourself. Don't ruin your peace. Don't smear yourself by creating a strict division between good and bad, vice and virtue. Have compassion, but not emotional involvement. Mind, you must find out how to do that.

Mind, let me create my own world. Let me adjust this external world the way I want. Let me overcome my delusion that things here are permanent. Let me correct my mistaken view that I am the owner of things in my possession and even of things not in my possession. Mind, remember that I am simply a guest in the courtyard of this great host called nature. This host delights in providing the best it has and gives in abundance what I can receive and retain. Blame no one—neither a person nor nature nor Providence. Such is the right view.

2. Right Resolve

To contemplate the means of making a right resolution regarding problems in your life, prepare your environment and compose yourself as you did for the first practice. Postpone worldly concerns and withdraw into yourself. This second step is meant to help you assimilate the theoretical knowledge that you have gained so far and to strengthen your determination to practice the higher values that you have abstracted from a spiritually grounded philosophy.

Recall an incident in which you did something which you knew at the time you should not have done, or taken a wrong action that you could have easily avoided. Recall the entire sequence of thoughts and events and contemplate:

How poor is my resolution, that in spite of knowing what is not right for me, and in spite of my decision not to do such things, I did this. Mind, it is due to the weakness of your resolution and determination. Mind, wake up, gather your strength. Remember and act.

This stage of contemplation is a means of acknowledging the stronger part of yourself and making the best use of it. Any sensible person knows what is right and what is wrong. At a conscious level, no one wants to get involved in an unhealthy and painful act. And yet, how easy it is to take such actions because of weak resolution and frail determination. By studying your own mind and heart and observing your strengths and weaknesses with the help of right resolution, you enable the stronger part of yourself to conquer the weaker part.

3. Right Speech

After establishing yourself in right views and right resolve, you must find the appropriate tools for expressing these views and this resolution. The first step in expressing right resolution is speech itself. Before our worldview and resolution can coalesce in action, it is reflected in our speech. A person who cannot discipline his or her speech will have a difficult time expressing his or her inner virtues through action. Speech is the coordination point between thought and action. It is the greatest vehicle of communication. Therefore, a person on the path of self-transformation should occasionally contemplate right speech:

How quickly words slip from my mouth. How easily my habits of speech permit me to forget my resolutions. How powerfully my words affect others. And how strongly others' words affect me.

During casual conversation, how much effort do I make to maintain my awareness of my philosophy of life and the higher values I have nurtured? How spontaneously and effortlessly my words express the contents of my mind. And in my effortless, spontaneous expression, what attitudes slip from my lips most often?

The predominant attitudes slipping from the mindfield through your speech reveal the contents of your mind. If the contents are not positive, creative, and healthy, then try to find some powerful antidotes—positive, creative, and healthy thoughts. These positive contents are also in the mind—it is simply a matter of unfolding these and raising them to the level of conscious awareness.

During your contemplation, recall instances in which you spoke in a manner that you regret. What were the emotional impulses behind this verbal outburst? This inner analysis of your habits of speech is a powerful means of studying your own thoughts and subtle behaviors, and thereby, of improving your relationships with yourself and others.

4. Right Conduct

Right resolve and right speech automatically lead to the performance of right action. But because our resolution is not always strong and we do not always control our tongues, it is necessary to pay attention to our actions. Day and night, a human being acts. There are no exact formulas for performing these actions, but by keeping the following five virtues in mind, we can learn to perform our actions skillfully and properly. The five virtues are: nonviolence, truthfulness, non-stealing, non-sensuality, and non-possessiveness.

It is important to spend a few minutes each day evaluating your actions and determining whether through

your actions you have harmed anyone. What was the
quality of your actions? How much lying, cunning, and
cheating were involved? How tenaciously did you grasp
your share? How many actions that appeared loving on
the surface were motivated by your sensual desires?
Which of your actions were driven by greed? When you
find your actions and behaviors relatively free of these
stains, reward your mind:

> **Thank you, Lord, for dwelling in my heart in the
> form of conscience and inspiring me to do only that
> which is right.**

When you find that some of your actions are causing
pain to others, involving you in lying or in taking what is
not yours, or are motivated by sense gratification or greed,
sit down and have a dialogue with your mind. But do not
condemn yourself; that will only weaken you. These are
simple mistakes made by every human who ever lived,
not unforgivable sins. Sit quietly and have a dialogue with
yourself:

> **Lord, give me strength and guide my mind and
> heart in the right direction. Let me be aware of the
> higher values of life which truly give me solace of
> heart. Let me acknowledge the tricks of my mind and
> my silly actions so that I may overcome them once
> and for all. Tell me, my Lord, why I forget the things**

I know and thus end up doing the things I don't want to do.

This stage of contemplation is very important because it will lead you to discover whether you are honest or hypocritical. The pitfall, however, is that we tend to create guilt and start condemning ourselves. Guilt and self-condemnation cripple inner strength and undermine self-confidence. Acknowledge your wrongdoings but do not judge. Find the flaws in your conduct and delight in your ability to discover these flaws. According to the yogic view, self-discovery is its own reward. This stage of contemplation enables you to discover your true image, whether it is positive or negative, and gives you the strength to transform yourself.

Self-transformation is more effective than working with a priest or a therapist. Self-transformation enables you to become honest with yourself and afterward, you do not care whether others acknowledge your honesty or not. Attain firm grounding in the principle of right conduct, and you will automatically understand the importance of right livelihood, the next step of the practice.

5. Right Livelihood

This contemplation requires an understanding of the basic law of life: whatever is born is granted food and shelter. All creatures—pigs and shrews, moles and tigers, elephants and sloths—find nourishment and refuge. But somehow humans no longer have a natural way of obtaining these things. Although humans can survive in any climate, so far they have not found a way of earning their livelihood while maintaining peace and harmony among themselves.

According to the scriptures, all domestic quarrels originate in the kitchen and center around food and drink, gradually spreading from there into other areas of family life. Unrest in a nation or among nations is also rooted in the quest for food, shelter, and other types of sustenance. The roots of cheating, stealing, and deception can be traced to how one makes one's living.

Many human beings fail to confine the idea of "making a living" to obtaining food and shelter. Some people are simply trying to meet their immediate physical needs; the "needs" of others are so immense that a billion dollars is not enough. In order to acquire more they will capture land, plunder the wealth of their neighbors, and even enslave others. Just as individuals are engrossed in "making a living," so are businesses, communities, and societies.

We each must contemplate the purity of our livelihoods. The best measure of "right livelihood" is the peace and harmony maintained while earning and enjoying your living. The less disturbance created in your own heart and in the lives of others, the more "right" your livelihood.

The following contemplation is a means of assimilating this principle and living with this truth:

Is my livelihood compatible with my worldview and my philosophy of life? Am I really happy with the work I do and the money I earn doing it? If not, is it just a mental habit of mine to be unhappy with whatever I do or is it the quality and effect of the work itself that makes me unhappy? Am I questioning my work because I don't get along with my co-workers or because I feel that I am underpaid? Or am I uneasy with the quality of the work itself?

Am I harming other beings in the course of earning my livelihood? Am I damaging the planet or creating pain or hostility in others? If so, is there any alternative? Am I sharing the fruits of my endeavor with those who are karmically connected with me? How balanced is my life in regard to what I accumulate? Am I really enjoying the fruits of my labor or am I overindulging myself? To what extent do I remain aware that all the objects of the world are simply meant to make my life comfortable and peaceful so that a greater amount of time and energy can be directed toward attaining the highest goal of life? Is my livelihood serving this purpose or has it become a goal in itself?

6. *Right Effort*

A person trying to live a balanced and harmonious life through right views, right resolve, right speech, right conduct, and right livelihood still faces the deeply rooted subtle impressions of past deeds, which play a significant role in daily life. Subtle impressions of the past that are stored in the unconscious mind motivate our conscious mind, senses, and body. As a result, there are times in life when we fail to do what we know is right. Powerful psychological and spiritual tools—methods of meditation, contemplation, and prayer, and a variety of breathing exercises—have been developed through the ages to conquer and transform these subtle tendencies hidden in the unconscious mind. All of these methods require effort. Nothing can be accomplished without work.

Each individual must decide which technique or combination of techniques will be most helpful—meditation, contemplation, prayer, study of the scriptures, the company of more evolved souls, or self-analysis. Applying the following process of contemplation will enable you to discern which particular techniques will best help you deal with the subtle tendencies in your unconscious mind.

Sit quietly, close your eyes, and ask yourself:

When I am not successful in the process of self-discovery and self-improvement, is it because I lack a clear understanding of my right view, right resolve,

right speech, right conduct, and right livelihood? Or am I clear about these issues but lose my balance and create a mess for myself because of my strong sense cravings? Or do my old habits and unknown subtle tendencies of my unconscious mind keep me from doing what I know is right? Am I too much influenced by my environment and the company I keep, and am therefore unable to organize myself and lead a healthy life? What is it that is stopping me from creating the kind of life I value?

If this process leads to the realization that your problems stem from confusion about right views, resolve, speech, conduct, and livelihood, then studying the texts, further contemplation, and the company of those who have a clearer knowledge of these things will all be helpful. If you notice that your problems are due to your uncontrolled sense cravings, then you need a systematic method of dealing with your body and mind. A discipline consisting of a balanced diet, exercise, deep yogic breathing, a schedule for going to bed and getting up, and gradual withdrawal from the objects of sense gratification will be helpful. If you are creating trouble for yourself with your habits, you need a systematic method of meditation. If your environment and companions are the source of your problems, the remedy lies in seeking the right environment and in living with people who are spiritually aware.

7. Right Mindfulness

You must keep your mind occupied with thoughts that are healthy for you and helpful to others. The mind is an energy field that cannot be emptied—it must contain thought constructs. If you do not deliberately supply it with healthy thoughts, then it pulls content directly from the bed of its memory without discrimination. If your storehouse of memories does not contain pleasant and spiritually elevating thoughts, you will end up thinking destructive thoughts that will wreak havoc in your life. An empty mind is the devil's playground. Before the devils have a chance to play their wild games, build the temple of the Divine so that the Divine can shine forth instead. Practicing the following contemplation, once or twice a day, even for a few minutes, will help purify the mind and fill it with joyful thoughts.

What are the thoughts that constantly and involuntarily occupy my mind and heart? Why do such thoughts come into my mind? How trivial they are, and yet I cling to them, thinking they are clinging to me. Mind, drop this delusion.

Another approach is to ask yourself:

Why, in spite of constantly cleaning my mind, does it still become filled with trash? . . . Oh, yes, it's

because I'm doing only half the job. I empty the mind, but because I do not fill it up again with positive thoughts, the trash comes back to fill the vacuum. Therefore, let me occupy my mind with constructive thoughts, remembering that the great masters of the past have said that constructive thoughts are twofold: constant awareness of the evanescent and trivial nature of worldly objects; and the knowledge that the purpose of life is Self-realization—not hand-to-mouth, office-to-bed existence. Therefore, mind, never forget that you are on an eternal journey. Don't get lost in the scenes you see. Keep the destination in mind.

Mind, in the procession of life, do not waste your time fighting with others and holding others back so you can get ahead. Walk on the path humbly, gently, and skillfully, with full focus only on the goal. Have compassion for those fellow travellers who surround you. Let them walk with you. If you have a better understanding of the map and the goal, humbly share your knowledge. If possible, give them a ride. And remember, at all costs, don't be confused by that foe, thoughts of distinction between "mine and not mine." Mind, allow me to always remember that I am on an eternal journey.

Thus, let the mind be filled with the awareness of the Supreme Goal. This is right mindfulness.

8. *Right Meditation*

Right meditation is a deepening of the contemplative truth practiced at the level of right mindfulness. Because the mind is accustomed to perceiving things with the senses, it is difficult for the mind to comprehend Truth, which is subtle, dissimilar to worldly objects, and does not come through the senses. Therefore, it is necessary to present a comprehensible idea of the Truth for the mind to grasp. It is for this reason that in different spiritual traditions, Truth is given different names and forms.

It is best not to superimpose many mundane characteristics on Truth, for such superimpositions are the basis of cultural and religious differences and thus are the source of strife. Because none of the symbols for Truth or God that have been invented by the human mind perfectly describes the nature of Truth, the yogic tradition prefers to avoid symbols or images. Yoga simply refers to the Truth as "Pure Consciousness." Pure existence, pure consciousness, and pure bliss are intrinsic to Truth. Or, as Buddhism expresses it, Truth is characterized by wisdom and compassion.

It is of utmost importance to meditate on the Truth using a system that carries the fewest possible cultural and religious biases. For example, light can be used as a symbol of Truth; meditating on light twice a day is a powerful means of keeping the mind focused on Truth. Meditating on the principles of love and compassion is also helpful, as it is in the kingdom of love and compassion that wisdom unfolds.

The Path of Meditation

The path of meditation is systematic and can be subdivided into three parts—concentration, meditation, and perfect spiritual absorption. The first step is to concentrate on the idea or principle itself—in this case, light or the principles of love or compassion. Before it is possible to resolve to concentrate on a principle, one must have an intense interest in it, which comes from understanding its value. Because of this zeal, the aspiring meditator attends to the idea itself, or to a teacher or to a book explaining it. The degree of attention determines how concentrated the mind is on that principle, which in turn determines how firmly it is grasped. A firm grasp and a burning desire to live with the principle enables the aspirant to retain it in his or her mind for a prolonged period.

Prolonged retention is the essence of meditation. The difference between concentration and meditation is the length of time the object of concentration is retained in the mind. If the mind retains the object for the time required to complete twelve inhalations and exhalations without another thought intervening, that is meditation. And when the mind is so absorbed for this twelve-breath period that it is not aware of anything at all, that is called perfect spiritual absorption (*samadhi*).

A Method of Meditation

Sit with your head, neck, and trunk straight. Place your hands comfortably either on your knees or in your lap. Withdraw your mind and senses from the external world. Mentally observe your body and the place occupied by your body. Once your body is still and your breath is steady, visualize a flame either in the area of your heart or at the point between your eyebrows. At the first glimpse of light in either of these two regions, offer your love and respect to that light as the representative of the highest truth within and without. Pay your homage: "Great Eternal Light, enlighten my path and the paths of all. May we all walk on the path of Truth without stumbling. Shine so brightly that we may see Thee even from this shore of life."

After paying this homage, let your mind focus on the light. The moment you notice that your mind is wandering, and therefore that your focus on the light has become unsteady, immediately resolve to bring your awareness back to the light.

Your concentration will be enhanced if you pay attention to your breath. While inhaling, imagine that you hear the sound "so," and without creating a pause, begin exhaling and hear the sound "hum." "So" simply means "that";

"hum" means "I am." Keep breathing and listening to the sound "so hum" with full awareness of its meaning, "I am that, I am that." As your awareness deepens, the meaning also expands and you may feel:

I am that Light, the Divine Light, I am that Light that shines in all individual hearts. I am that Light which is the purest and the most accurate image of the Supreme Lord, the Almighty.

I am that Light. My true essence is that Light, not the physical appearance that I carry all the time. There may be differences in our external appearances, but deep down, we are one and the same. All living beings are pure Light. That Light alone is life. Let me honor that life. Let that Light enlighten my life and the lives of all. Peace, Peace, Peace.

The Fruit of Practice

This eightfold path of contemplation, which culminates in meditation on Truth, makes the mind one-pointed and purifies the heart, filling it with love and compassion. Nonviolence flows spontaneously from such a heart.

Once we, as individuals, are established in the principle of nonviolence, our society will no longer be ruled so completely by fear and greed. We will no longer need police forces or armies. Free from all enemies, we finally will attain freedom from the most implacable enemy of all—war itself.

This ideal state of nonviolence represents the highest stage of human evolution. Although we have not yet evolved to such a sublime state of consciousness, there is power in visualizing ourselves at this pinnacle. If we long for peace, we must aspire to it. To attain it, we must set to work with great energy. That is the only way we will ever free ourselves from both the war within and the war without.

Two

Like a lotus that grows from the mud and blooms above the water, rise beyond your little pond, blossom, and let the world partake of your fragrance.

Nonviolence:
The Antidote to War

I n the yogic tradition, the word for "nonviolence" is *ahimsa*. The literal meaning of *ahimsa* is "not hurting, non-killing, or not damaging." But none of these phrases accurately captures the profundity of the concept of *ahimsa*. *Ahimsa* (which I will translate as "nonviolence" in the interest of brevity), connotes "non-harmfulness" at every level of existence. There are philosophical, ideological, and spiritual injuries, as well as physical, verbal, and psychological injuries. *Ahimsa* connotes nonviolence at all these levels simultaneously.

Manifestations of Violence

T he most obvious violence is physical violence. A person becomes violent and hurts others under certain psychological conditions—every violent person is psychologically ill, at least at the moment of violence. Physical violence is the outer manifestation of the subtle violence that we carry within and usually fail to acknowledge.

In some ways, physical violence is easier to contend with than verbal or psychological violence, and can actually be less damaging. Physical abuse is palpable and its effects are immediately visible. Therefore, it is likely to be brief. The person committing the violence immediately notices what he or she is doing, and often realizes the mistake; this realization is usually enough to snap him or her back to a quasi-normal state. If not, then someone else often intervenes. But because verbal violence is less tangible, it will probably continue longer. Furthermore, physical violence harms the body, but verbal violence affects a deeper level of being—the mind, the emotions, and the spirit. In a verbal fight, both parties are injured, and the effects are long lasting. The wounds inflicted in a physical fight can be treated with antiseptics and bandages, but the wounds inflicted by speech are not so visible and cannot be so easily treated. If the verbal injury is not treated immediately, an infection begins that sooner or later will erupt in more violence.

Verbal violence is rooted in mental violence. Before we hurt others with our speech, there must be a violent thought in the mind. Such violent thoughts are the result, not of intellectual analysis or proper thinking, but rather of our emotional outbursts, which momentarily override the faculty of discrimination. In most situations, we react on the basis of our emotional impulses. As long as our reactions are discerned and restrained by the faculty of discrimination, we behave peaceably; but if our emotional reactions are not screened by the discriminative faculty, we behave wildly. The problem is exacerbated when our emotions are controlled, not by wisdom but by another emotion—fear of being punished, for example, or the desire to stay on good terms with someone in power. Repressed emotions are the ground for mental violence, and in this fertile soil, verbal and physical violence germinate.

Violence at a psychological level originates in the form of a negative thought, such as hatred, anger, jealousy, or the desire for revenge. If this negative thought does not find expression, the person holding it becomes volatile. Negative thoughts are painful, and without a healthy means of expressing them, the thinker remains in pain. Due to a lack of self-knowledge, such a person will not understand why he or she is so unhappy and will seek an outside cause. At the merest excuse, this person will accuse someone else of causing his or her troubles. If the other person denies the accusation, a verbal battle ensues. Unresolved, this verbal conflict can escalate into a physical altercation or even a war.

Violence also takes philosophical or ideological forms. People who are fully convinced that their ideas are the only authentic ideas may not only attempt to impose them everywhere, but may also vehemently condemn the ideas of others. This is often seen in disputes between two scholars, philosophers, or teachers. A religious crusade is an example of ideological violence, as are disputes over political and economic systems such as communism and capitalism.

Spiritual violence is also common. Taking the Truth for granted, spiritual teachers sometimes misguide their followers. In a sense, this is spiritual violence. In this particular area, giving a specific example could cause great offense, which would in itself be a form of violence. That is why, in the realm of spirituality, silence is often considered to be the best policy.

The Animal, the Human, and the Divine

All forms of violence are common among human beings. But this is not ordained—violence among humans is not inevitable. Far from being an intrinsic part of our nature, as is commonly assumed, violence is an aberration.

According to the scriptures, every human being is born with three qualities—animal, human, and divine. During infancy and early childhood, all three tendencies manifest, and all three seek an environment in which to grow and find expression. Because there is a divine being, a human being, and an animal within each individual, a baby can be raised as a sage, as a gentle loving human, or as a criminal. Through proper training, education, and loving guidance, the beast within can be transformed first into a pet and then into a human. The same human can later expand his or her consciousness and become divine.

If the parents have not freed themselves from the negative forces of attachment, anger, hatred, jealousy, greed, and fear and thus do not care for higher virtues, such as selflessness, love, compassion, and generosity, then the animal tendencies will be strengthened in the child they rear. If the parents nourish these animal tendencies, the child will grow outwardly as a human, but internally as an animal, and will exhibit animal behavior as an adult. Although this being may not have a tail and horns or walk on all fours, in terms of behavior, such a human differs little from the members of the animal kingdom.

The scriptures say that humans and animals have four qualities in common—the four primitive urges of hunger, sleep, sex, and fear (or the desire for self-preservation). All emotions spring from these four primitive urges. The degree of control one has over these emotions marks a being as either human or animal. Fear and hunger seem to be the most dominant of the four primitive urges. Animals devote most of their energy avoiding their predators and searching for food.

Although all four urges play a key role in the lives of humans, in most cases, the faculty of discrimination serves to balance their effect on our actions. Much of our behavior is controlled neither by these urges nor by the emotions they generate. To some extent, we have the capacity to subordinate our individual urges to the needs of others. But if we allow these urges to drive our behavior, they will consume us and we will become self-serving, defensive, and fearful. These are animal tendencies. Rising above such tendencies—by cultivating concern for others and deepening our sensitivity to the needs of others, even in the face of self-serving urges—elevates us from animal to human. From here, we can unfold the higher virtues of selfless love and compassion, and move toward the Divine. But we can become divine only after we have become fully human.

The Genesis of Fear

According to yoga tradition, the process of training and taming the animal within and transforming it into a human and then into the Divine is accomplished by the practice of nonviolence. The power of nonviolence to so transform a human can be understood by examining the relationship between violence and fear, and between nonviolence and fearlessness.

Fear of death is the greatest of all fears. All other fears are pale shadows of this primal terror. Fear of death is innate to anything that is born—a human, an animal, an insect, or even a plant. Every living being has developed defense mechanisms in response to this inborn fear. Other species focus more of their energy on developing their defense mechanisms than do humans. This, according to yoga, is because they are consumed by fear. In humans, there are many other tendencies balancing the survival instinct.

Seeking to understand fear, the yogis searched for a cause and found twins—attachment and aversion. A human being forms a more powerful bond with family members and pleasing objects than do other animals. And this strong attachment to some people and things automatically results in aversion to other people and things. Humans constantly strive to achieve what they like and to rid themselves of what they dislike. Furthermore, it is usually a personal sense of liking and disliking, rather than need, that makes us characterize an object as good or bad. Humans are afraid of not getting what they want and of ending up with things they do not want.

Because humans are highly developed beings, their wants, desires, likes, and dislikes are legion. Therefore, the sources of their fears are more numerous than those of other, less-evolved species. One facet of evolution is the development of a self-identity—the sense of "I-am-ness" discussed earlier.

A human being is a conglomerate of numberless identities. Each individual's sense of "I-am-ness" contains myriad elements—good, bad, healthy, strong, rich, poor, Hindu, Moslem, American, European, wife, husband, son, daughter, and so on. Within each of these identities, an individual carries an enormous burden of likes and dislikes, attachments and aversions. Each element of this burden creates a fear that some part of the identity will be lost or taken away or that an unwanted identity will be imposed.

All fear can be traced to attachment and aversion, and attachment and aversion can be traced to self-identity—"I-am-ness," or ego. Our inclination to defend or attack has its genesis in our fear of losing something that we believe to be integral to our identity. Just as pain is a symptom of disease, violence is a symptom of fear. Fever counters threats from a virus or bacteria, and violence counters threats to identity. Fever and violence are both indications of an internal struggle. An uncontrolled fever can jeopardize life, as can violence. As long as there is fear and the cause for fear, violence will recur. The more fearless we are, the more nonviolent we become.

The freer a person is from fear, the more open that person is. A fearful person is sealed in his or her own little world and, as a result, suffers from emptiness and loneliness. But a person who is free from fear is open and loving. Such a person has minimized his or her attachment and aversion, and so is naturally less caught in the idea of losing and gaining and is thus free of stress and tension. Such a person remains tranquil in all situations.

The Cycle of Violence

When nonviolent instincts are overridden by negative, violent forces, a human becomes even more dangerous than creatures in the wild. Fortunately, such an occurrence is relatively rare—only a fraction of humanity cripples its human virtues by nourishing the violent tendencies of the animal within. Violence is an aberration, and all societies have methods of isolating overtly violent individuals from the rest of us.

Humans are usually nonviolent. Even hurting or killing our enemies is something we normally avoid. And yet, others make these decisions on our behalf. The question is, who are these others? Are they really so different from us? Are they not our representatives? As our representatives, they must represent what we feel in some way. At some level, we are all involved in violence. At some level, we seek it and delight in it; otherwise, war and bloodshed would not be so widespread.

Violence cannot be abolished by assigning the blame to someone else. We can stop it only by examining our own thoughts and feelings. Human beings are masters of self-deception. To avoid listening to the voice of our own hearts, to lighten the burden of guilt, and to justify our inhumane deeds, we find grand and distancing words to describe our actions. For example, we use the word "casualty" to refer to a maimed or slaughtered human. According to psychologists, such words allow us to remain comfortable with descriptions of violence. The terms "collateral damage," and "carpet bombing" are other examples. These words are used to soften the facts so that civilians don't become frantic and demand an end to the violence.

The point of describing our adroitness at deceiving ourselves is that we must acknowledge our violent tendencies and their bloody consequences. Denying our destructive tendencies or hiding them with sweet-sounding words will not change them. As long as the root of violence remains, it will find expression.

We must stop pretending that it is possible to end war and violence with war and violence. Short of a nuclear holocaust, there can be no "war to end all wars." The past has shown us that the seeds of the wars to come are planted in the current war. The mind has a penchant for remembering the event but forgetting the lesson. We must train our minds to remember the lessons and somehow forget the events. The memory of the events evokes the irrational causes behind them; thus the perpetrators of irrational acts are never forgiven. And because in any war, each side considers the other to be the irrational perpetrator, the stage is set for the next act of destruction.

The Power of Nonviolence

Nonviolence is the only constructive strategy for engaging

the enemy. Before, during, and after its application, it remains non-destructive and non-painful. Nonviolence is the only weapon that renders B-52 bombers, Scud missiles, and "Smart" weapons impotent. Practitioners of nonviolence are the only soldiers who attain ultimate victory. Nonviolence is the only force that transforms an enemy into a friend: the winner surrenders to the loser, the loser to the winner, and both attain victory.

This superior method of doing battle has been employed several times in the past; each time it led to victory. The practice of nonviolence begins with individuals and because "similar attracts similar," it spreads, pervading the community, then the nation, and finally the entire human race. It is a slow process but a sure one. It is long-lasting and has no adverse side effects.

People often argue that we need a leader like Buddha, Christ, or Gandhi to initiate a war of nonviolence. A yogi would respond that there is a Buddha, a Christ, and a Gandhi in each individual heart. A part of every individual is as enlightened, merciful, compassionate, loving, and fearless as Buddha, Christ, or Gandhi. Such souls incarnate at the call of the compassionate and nonviolent forces within us.

Each time we call, a Buddha emerges among us. The Bible says, "Ask, and it will be given." But the Bible doesn't specify what to ask for and therefore what will be given. A collective consciousness asked for Saddam Hussein and got him. A collective consciousness called for George Bush and he's there.

We get whatever we ask for. God Almighty is immeasurably generous, but He must shudder when we silly children ask for knives to cut our fingers. God has nothing to do with what we do to ourselves. We can use the gifts, the grace, and the intelligence that have been granted us for either right or wrong. We often use it for wrong, sharpening our intellect and using it to exploit nature and each other for selfish ends.

This is where we violate the principle of nonviolence. Possessiveness and nonviolence are incompatible; nonviolence walks hand-in-hand with selflessness. Hatred and violence, love and nonviolence, giving and receiving, accepting others and being accepted by others—these are perfect pairs. Knowing this and living in the light of this knowledge is the key to nonviolence.

Nonviolence must be practiced before and after a war, as well as while it is going on. In fact, practitioners of nonviolence can accomplish more after a war than they can while it is raging. A practitioner of nonviolence studies the nature and movement of the magma that builds up during the time of "peace," and finds way to drain and cool it. A proponent of nonviolence knows that a peace that is only the gap between two wars is a superficial peace. Deep beneath this peaceful surface, hatred, anger, greed, ego, possessiveness, and the desire for revenge brew and seethe. During the gap between two wars, nations and factions race to build or acquire arms—a race that is simply preparation for the next war.

During wartime, when the volcano is erupting, it is almost impossible to practice and teach nonviolence. In the midst of war, people are obsessed with winning the war or escaping its consequences. It is during the period of peace that the real work of fostering nonviolence can be done. During a war, providing food, medical care, and money will save lives and ameliorate the immediate suffering, but cultivating the power of nonviolence during the interval of peace, will spare future generations the immense physical and emotional damage that attends war.

The power of nonviolence is beyond the grasp of an ordinary mind. Darkness cannot face the brilliance of nonviolence. If the human race is ever to coalesce into a harmonious society of peaceful nations, it will do so on the firm ground of nonviolence and selfless love. But mere belief in the principles of nonviolence is not sufficient. Even now, most people in the world believe in nonviolence, but wars still rage. This is because nonviolence is an abstract principle to most of us, a passive belief rather than an active part of our lives. Making it active requires living it in thought, speech, and action.

Just as soldiers are trained in the precise methods of finding and striking military targets, so are there precise methods of practicing nonviolence and targeting the injured areas of our lives at both the individual and the collective level. Skillful use of nonviolence requires that we overcome our violent tendencies within and without. These techniques bear no resemblance to the practices in psychiatric institutions where violent people are rendered inert with drugs and other methods. There is nothing inert about nonviolence. It is a demanding way of life, supported by a sound philosophy and fueled by spiritual practice.

Becoming Nonviolent: Nine Contemplative Practices

If practiced sincerely, the following contemplations will create a firm grounding in the principles of nonviolence. These practices will enable us to transform ourselves and to gain a better understanding of ourselves, our friends, and our "enemies." They will also help us to cultivate a positive worldview and sound philosophy of life. In the initial stages of this practice, participants will benefit individually and the influence will gradually spread.

The sages of the past have promised that when you become peaceful and happy, love and compassion will radiate from you. People will bask in your light and warmth and will wonder why you are so pleasant and loving. This curiosity will lead them to observe your lifestyle and ask about your philosophy. They will want to know your secret, and because the secret is so simple—don't hurt yourself and don't hurt others—they will begin to emulate you. And that is how the power of nonviolence emerges from the heart of individuals and begins to pervade the family, community, and society. One day it will surely pervade the whole human race. But first, individuals—you and me—must begin practicing the principle of nonviolence systematically. This is not a religious commandment; we must not impose this principle on others. This is not a business strategy; there is no need to penetrate the market. This principle is a nectar, and wherever there is nectar, honeybees gather. Nectar sends a silent invitation to all honeybees. Let us begin to gather it.

1. Do Not Kill Your Conscience

We kill our consciences when we continue to do things we do not want to do while postponing the things we want to do. Working against the conscience creates an internal battle—the inner self is split, each part warring with the other. Once this inner conflict is underway, your mind becomes utterly confused. The confused mind wavers back and forth between right and wrong, just and unjust, without establishing a firm ground anywhere.

People with confused minds are vulnerable to emotional appeals and can be swayed by sensational speeches. They become entranced by demagogues and tend to join mass movements without giving much consideration to whether or not the cause is good or just. If the cause is unjust and they come to realize it, they feel guilty. Guilt leads to self-condemnation, which in turn perpetuates the process of killing the conscience.

The practice of nonviolence begins with cultivating the conscience. Once the seed of nonviolence has been sown in the conscience, truth will sprout. The first step in cultivating the conscience is to take time to listen to the voice of your heart. Periodically, once a week if possible, put aside all opinions regarding disturbances in the external world—such as international crises; political controversies; or conflicts at work, in the community, or with your family. If your nation is at war, try to find time for this practice every day. For five minutes, drop all thoughts of enemy, friend, nationality, race, or gender from your mind. Find yourself on common ground with your opponent—both of you are humans. Holding that perspective, try to discern what your relations are with your opponent and how balanced your reactions are. Listen to the voice of your heart, the voice of the soul, which has equal love and concern for both of you. Your heart will tell you what is right.

When you hear the voice of your heart, don't allow your mind to become frightened. Mind is accustomed to being selfish, egotistical, and skeptical. Just as one army disrupts the radio transmissions of another by jamming them with extraneous noise, so the mind transmits static to garble the voice of the heart. Do not allow your mind to create interference. The fewer noises created by your mind, the clearer the voice of your heart. The clearer the voice of your heart, the closer you are to Truth. The fewer fears you have of losing your selfish objectives, the longer you will retain the light of Truth. A burning desire for Truth and reverence for life itself will help you create the environment where you can contemplate these matters.

2. Do Not Condemn Another's Way of Life

Differences in geography, terrain, vegetation, climate, and natural resources engendered different ways of life. Studies by anthropologists and philologists show that to a great extent each culture's religion, philosophy, customs, superstitions, and other values are shaped by these factors. Viewed from this perspective, every way of life has its own reason for being and its own integrity. We make a mistake when we use our own cultural standards to judge the values of another culture. For example, we consider cultures with fewer material objects—automobiles, televisions, telephones, and indoor plumbing—to be "poor." Similarly, we call a person who is unfamiliar with our convoluted economic system and our complex technological society "ignorant." In both cases, such people may be richer and wiser than we are, in terms of contentment, honesty, truthfulness, peace, and happiness.

One of the main causes of violence is the tendency to label others and pass judgements on their way of life, especially when this is done with the intention of imposing our ideas, value systems, and lifestyles on them. Even if it is done with the best of intentions, an adverse reaction is inevitable. Every community identifies itself with a set of social, cultural, and religious values, developing an attachment for them that often borders on reverence. Challenging these values is tantamount to challenging the identity, the sense of "I-am-ness" of every member of the community. Those so challenged will respond with fear and anger.

The failure to understand that others' values are as important to them as ours are to us breeds intolerance. Tolerance is the cushion that absorbs the shock of our mutual differences and once that cushion is gone, the impact can be brutal. In the absence of tolerance, the impulses that lead to violence thrive.

Tolerance is integral to nonviolence. The following contemplation is one way of assimilating this principle:

Look at the diversity in the world. Certainly it is part of nature. If diversity were not natural, then God would have designed all the mountains in the same fashion. All humans would have the same faces. People everywhere would have the same skin tone. But how boring and redundant that would be. It is the same with lifestyle and values—it is natural for humans to express their diversity in that way too.

Let me not condemn how others think and what

they think. It doesn't matter whether or not their values are profound and meaningful to me. Let me learn to respect them and their beliefs exactly the way I want others to respect me and mine.

3. Do Not Label Others

This is an expansion of the suggestion to refrain from condemning the way of life of others. The concepts of virtue and vice, merits and demerits that we nourish in our minds, cloud our vision. We forget that most values are conventional, and subject to time and place. That which seems virtuous today might not seem virtuous tomorrow. Similarly, a particular method of worshipping God which seems elevating in one culture may seem silly or barbaric in another.

We have a tendency to categorize individuals by identifying them with certain groups, and then attributing a blanket set of characteristics to that group. Thus, we make such statements as, "These Americans always . . .," " Arabs never. . .," "Buddhists usually . . .," or "South Africans don't . . . ." That is how we create prejudices in our mind and jump to conclusions about others on the basis of partial or erroneous information. Sweeping generalizations are absurd at best and dehumanizing at worst: not all beings in the Himalayas are sages; not all Americans are decadent; not all Moslems are seeking martyrdom; and not all prison guards are brutal.

Although many prejudices are subtle, they manifest in our thoughts, speech, and actions. Often we fail to notice them at all, or if we do, we may not consider them to be significant. But when the time comes to interact with other groups or to make decisions regarding them, these subtle traces of our prejudices surface and prevent us from seeing these "others" in their full complexity and humanness.

Violence has its roots in prejudice and the habit of creating labels. When one group dehumanizes another by applying pernicious labels, war is imminent. Often this is done deliberately to make the "enemy" seem as alien as possible so that killing him or her will be less appalling.

The following contemplation is one means of eradicating the tendency to label and dehumanize others:

How can I judge the children of God whom he created in his own image? Let me not label any of God's images and discriminate against them because to do so shows disrespect for the Creator. Let me examine the purity of my own heart instead. Let me observe how skillfully I refrain from cultivating prejudices against those who do not belong to my religion, faith, creed, and culture.

Let me remember that we are all children of God and that each person is an individual, just as I am. And let me refrain from harming anyone through my thoughts, words, or action, no matter how different from me they seem.

4. Do Not Preserve the Trash Deposited by History

The human race is divided into sundry groups, each with a sense of its own history. Just as calamities make newspaper headlines, the events most likely to be recorded in the history books are the dramatic, emotion-provoking episodes. And history, like every other area of life, is subject to interpretation and manipulation. So far, there is no complete or accurate history of any group or series of events. We end up studying partial histories and projecting the selective version of recorded events into the present and the future.

As a result of remembering and studying their various histories, Hindus, Jews, Moslems, and Christians have nourished ill-will toward each other. We recall and recount events of the past and try to punish the descendants of those we believe oppressed our ancestors. This is folly. We must learn to forget the events while remembering the lessons of those events. Let the historians pursue their research; let them dispute one anothers' findings, and argue about who did what to whom and whether or not it was justified. But for our own good, the rest of us should close the sad and vengeful chapters of the past to prevent them from poisoning the present. This is the only way to free ourselves from the anguish and vengeance passed down from generation to generation.

Instead of pondering over the injustices of the past,

whether real or imagined, let us contemplate:

> We all are members of the same species. We live on the same planet, consuming the same food and water, breathing the same air, and walking in the light of the same sun. We fight over the same things because we all are human and share the same hunger, thirst, and fear. How sad it is that we remember only the wars and other disputes and forget the good things we share and the feelings we have in common.
>
> It is a tendency of the human mind to keep careful track of negative, destructive, violent activities and spare barely a moment's thought for the good things. We must reverse this tendency and learn to retain only the good memories and let the trash be swept away.
>
> Let me find a way to do this, no matter what others do. Let me transform myself and let me change my habit of remembering the specifics regarding my family, clan, and race, especially in relation to people I have formed a habit of disliking and those who I believe dislike me.

5. Do Not Let Conventional Values Override Love, Compassion, and Nonviolence

Within the confines of a single community, whose people share common religious, cultural, and economic values, it is necessary to honor those values. However, it is important both to recognize that many of our values are conditioned by time and place and to honor the values of other communities, even when they are radically different from our own.

The values of universal love, compassion, and nonviolence are perennial and supersede all other values. If conventional values conflict with these universal values, the universal values take precedence. Conventional values are the means of maintaining law, order, and harmony within communities, but the higher values of love, compassion, and nonviolence are the means of bringing these smaller communities into a bigger fold. These higher values are the means of expanding our consciousness and teaching ourselves to focus on the interests of all humanity rather than centering our attention on the narrow interests of the group with which we identify. Here is how to contemplate this point:

I am a human—that is my primary identity. How can I subordinate my human identity and the human identity of others to the secondary identities of gender, ethnicity, nationality, religion, and

political philosophy?

Do not let my likes and dislikes, my attachments and aversions toward these secondary identities obscure the virtues of love, compassion, and nonviolence. Let me remember that, no matter how it may appear, the similarities between me and every other human in the world far outstrip the superficial differences.

6. *Individuals Are an Integral Part of the Same Organism*

All entities are interdependent. All beings, including all humans, are interconnected at one level or another. Although it may seem that we live independent lives, this independence is supported by a larger interdependence. This is apparent in the international community. For example, one nation's economy influences the economy of many other nations. The global communications network has made all members of the human race much more familiar with each other than we ever were in the past. It is no longer possible to hide either our richness or our poverty, our love or our hatred, or our good or bad intentions toward each other. It is becoming clear that all humans are part of a single global organism and it is crucial that we learn to act and communicate in perfect peace and harmony. Unrest in any enclave immediately spreads across the globe.

If we grind our teeth in our sleep and wake up with a headache, we don't destroy our teeth in order to teach them a lesson. Instead, we recognize that this behavior is a symptom of internal stress and set out to find the cause and the cure. So it should be in the outer world. Just as we grind our teeth in our sleep for a reason, there must be a reason why a segment of humanity causes pain to the rest. Any outward expression of violence is a symptom of internal stress. Instead of condemning the members of a group for being violent and either punishing or destroying them, it is better to find and uproot the cause of the violence.

One way of removing the source of stress is to find a better way of understanding and communicating with each other. Just as all organs of the body must function together in perfect coordination to ensure the health and well-being of the organism, all segments of the human community must work together to promote the well-being of humanity. If the mouth keeps food for itself, if the heart collects and hoards blood, if the lungs capture and stockpile air, the body is doomed.

The same is true of the organism of humanity. The major international problems—poverty, pollution, and political unrest—come into being because one part of the organism treats another part like an alien being. We forget that others are an integral part of ourselves and unwittingly enfeeble ourselves by weakening others and depriving them of their share. The following contemplation is a means of assimilating this knowledge:

> How am I connected with others, and how am I separate? Can I really exist apart from those who seem to be physically separate from me? Can humanity exist apart from humans and or humans from humanity? Not at all.
>
> There is a forest and there are trees in the forest. Are the trees completely different from the forest? It doesn't seem so. All the trees and shrubs—small and big, green and dry, those that bear fruit and those that are barren—make up the forest. If each tree and shrub is separated and removed, the forest no longer exists.
>
> It is the same with humans and humanity. And yet, how profound is our ignorance that believes we can damage the trees without harming the forest. Let me love all and live with the knowledge that everyone is part of me and that I am part of everyone.

7. There is Only One Lifeforce

Although we may be able to live separately at the physical level, one lifeforce runs through us all. This lifeforce sustains every aspect of existence—the world of minerals as well as the kingdom of plants, animals, and humans. All sentient beings need food, air, water, light, and heat. These elements have no preferences about who they nourish. They simply serve as vehicles of life energy, and in doing so, create a greater bond among us than we commonly realize.

The air we inhale travels through every cell of our bodies, gathers not only the toxins, but also thoughts and feelings, returns to the lungs, and is exhaled through our nostrils. All that we know at the deepest level of our being passes into the air outside our bodies. That air is then inhaled and assimilated into the systems of others, where the same process occurs again. Those who have developed their higher sensibilities experience the thoughts and feelings of others simply by coming into contact with the air in the atmosphere around them. Such is the nature of our existence and the depth of our mutual sharing.

By polluting or purifying our minds and hearts, we affect others. By affecting others, ultimately we affect ourselves. We can blind ourselves to this truth, but we cannot change it. According to the sages, whatever we do to others will be done to us—we reap what we sow. Hurting others is hurting ourselves; loving others is loving ourselves. There is no difference between us; the same lifeforce animates us all. A person who wants the love, respect, and honor of others must love, respect, and honor others.

It is obvious that a single force endows all beings with life. This single lifeforce sustains us all in its

dazzling diversity. I know this, and yet somehow I fail to see myself as an integral part of creation.

Why do I act as though I'm blind to the unity that underlies every aspect of existence? Let me love all in the full knowledge that loving all means loving myself because, under the surface, there is no difference between me and all other beings.

8. Hurting Anyone Means Hurting God

According to each of the world's great spiritual traditions, all individuals are children of God. From early childhood, we have heard the phrases, "All men are brothers," "Love thy neighbor as thyself," and "We are all God's children." Yet still we condemn and injure others. Just as parents are saddened when their children fight and injure each other, so must God be saddened watching us hurt one another. Remembering that hurting any of God's children is tantamount to hurting God will help us remember to treat one another with kindness and love. The following contemplation is helpful:

Mind, cast off your selfishness; it allows you to injure others. If you claim to love God, then you must not disappoint Him by hurting those whom He loves. You must not dishonor Him by dishonoring those whom He adores. He loves and adores, not only me, but every woman, man, and child on the face of the earth. By showing love to all His children, I show my love for God.

9. The Law of the Divine is the Only Auspicious Law

Law and order are necessary if humans are to live together in groups. Laws and other rules governing behavior vary from culture to culture and even among groups within one culture. When making rules and setting standards for behavior, we must be careful to define the boundaries of our group and to respect the boundaries of other groups. In the scriptures, the ground for performing one's duties is called *karma ksetra*. Just as there are individuals, societies, communities, and nations, so are there individual, communal, societal, and national "fields of duty." People may experience internal conflict when one field of duty overlaps and contradicts another. For example, the mother of a baby may find her individual field of duty in conflict with her societal and national fields of duty if she is also a soldier and her country is at war.

External conflicts arise when, in the performance of duty, one individual's or group's field of action intersects with that of another. Most of our troubles arise when we believe that the performance of our duty requires us to interfere with others who are performing their duties.

When this occurs at the group level, war is often the result. It is extremely difficult to know whether or not this interference is really necessary, although justifications can usually be found. This problem cannot be solved by the intellect alone. Intuitive wisdom, grounded in love, compassion, mutual understanding, and nonviolence is the best means of knowing whether or not we should intervene in the lives of other individuals, communities, societies, or nations. Because our intuitive wisdom is often buried under our selfishness, ego, fear, and attachment to our own conventional values, we often intervene when we should not and create turmoil for ourselves and others.

It is even difficult to contemplate this point, because without repeated practice in overcoming ego, selfishness, attachment, and aversion it is impossible to even see the problem. But we can pray to a higher power or to the Divinity within to give us the strength and wisdom to overcome our blindness so that we can walk in the light of divine law.

God, give me the wisdom to see that others have duties just as I have. Let me learn to be wary of my tendency to believe it is my duty to interfere with others. Before acting, let me always stop and examine whether the impulse to intervene springs from ego, fear, or attachment to my own values or from compassion and selfless love. Lead me to the sublime state of consciousness where I know, through my

own direct experience, that my true family is the human race. Let me embrace all and exclude none.

May I learn to delight in sacrificing my personal pleasures for the sake of my family. May I learn to sacrifice my family interests for the welfare of the community, and may I find the wisdom to sacrifice my communal interests for the welfare of my society. May I envision the ways of contributing to the welfare of the entire humanity, even if I have to sacrifice the welfare of "my" society.

Three

*To find the east, you need no ladder to scale the
horizon. The sun itself introduces the east.*

When War is Inevitable

War has been so pervasive throughout the ages and across the globe that it sometimes appears to be a universal principle. There are times when war seems inevitable and there are times when it seems a duty, although much depends on the angle of perception. Even if a particular war is inevitable or just or both, killing one's enemies runs counter to a basic tenet voiced by all of the world's great spiritual traditions. A few examples are Christ's urging to "Love your enemies;" the commandment "Thou shalt not kill," that God passed to the Jews through Moses, and the yogic exhortation to practice *ahimsa*.

Justifications for war have always accompanied war. Through the centuries these justifications have coalesced into a set of principles and have found their way into international law. According to these principles, in order for a war to be just it must be declared as a last resort by a "legitimate authority," and then only to support a just cause. Wars of aggression are never justified, although international law recognizes the legitimacy of wars waged to counter grave threats to international order or those joined on behalf of a helpless third party.

Although all of these justifications seem reasonable at first glance, they do not bear close scrutiny. What some call a "legitimate authority," others will call an outlaw government. What one nation views as a just cause, another nation will view as an outrage. And the "last resort" may never be reached because it is always possible to convene another round of talks. All of these points are controversial and subject to intellectual and emotional argument. For every person espousing one view, there is someone eager to refute it. Furthermore, none of these justifications can assuage grief. Philosophical arguments are cold comfort to those who have been maimed, or who have lost their loved ones, livelihood, or peace of mind as the result of war.

Like other philosophical and spiritual systems, yoga has grappled with the question of when war is justified. The sages recognized that when the forces of violence and destruction seize power, war may offer the only solution. But even then, it is almost impossible to sort through the options objectively and to be certain that taking up arms is the correct choice.

The mind is tricky and loath to know itself. Even the most conscientious thinker is prone to unconsciously twist ideas and facts to suit a preconceived notion or to justify a preferred course of action. Making the correct decision about whether or not war is necessary and justified requires profound analysis and scrupulous self-study. Those with whom the decision rests must exercise discrimination, listen to the voice of conscience, and analyze the facts honestly.

According to yoga, even if this painstaking process leads to a decision to declare war, the opponent must still be given many opportunities to back down. The scriptures say that if war is imminent because of domestic issues and both parties are part of the same family, then the wise man must forgive his opponent one hundred times before using military force.

These scriptures were written several thousand years ago, when monarchs ruled and kingdoms were inherited. Wars were fought over possession of the throne and often involved brothers. Although the particulars are different today, the essence is unchanged—the drive for power and possessions and the agony and chaos that attend war are the same in any century. In the third century BCE, *The Bhagavad Gita*, the great yoga scripture, tackled the question of when war is justified. According to legend, the profound wisdom of the *Gita* was imparted between the front lines of two opposing armies moments before a great battle. The following translation and interpretation of a portion of this text and its exposition of when and why fighting a war becomes one's duty provides a sense of the complexity of this problem.

The Road to War

The *Gita* is a dialogue between two great warriors. In order to place the dialogue in context, it is necessary to know something about the events preceeding it.

There once was a king who had a blind brother. In his early youth, this king entrusted his kingdom to his brother and retired to the forest with his wife and children. He died soon afterward, and the queen returned to the court with five sons. These children and the children of the blind regent were raised and educated together as brothers. But when the oldest son of the rightful king reached manhood and was ready to assume the throne, trouble began. The blind uncle was reluctant to step down. The rightful heir, who was generous and peace-loving, agreed to let him keep the throne for the remainder of his life. But that only fed the uncle's greed, and he hatched plots to ensure his own son's succession.

The blind regent and his sons made several attempts on the lives of the rightful heir and his four brothers, and things went from bad to worse. Scheme followed scheme, but throughout it all, the rightful ruler refused to resort to violence. Finally the wicked uncle and cousins contrived to exile the five brothers to the forest for thirteen years.

During this period of exile, the false king and his sons gathered an enormous military force, stockpiled weapons, and formed alliances with neighboring countries. Their subjects were miserable—taxes were heavy, with every penny used to increase the strength of the army; corruption was rampant; and women and children were not protected. People were praying for the rightful king and his four brothers to return from exile. When they did, the rightful king sent an emissary to the court with a proposal for getting his kingdom back. The emissary was mistreated and the proposal spurned.

Finally, Krishna, a man of the highest wisdom and a great king in his own right, undertook to settle the dispute. He went to the court of the wicked king with another peaceful proposal. This proposal was also scorned. Undaunted, the five brothers made yet another attempt, sending Krishna to say that they would be content with one village apiece, but the king and his eldest son refused to yield even a pinpoint of land without a fight. And so it went for several years, with Krishna and the five brothers trying to find a peaceful way to restore law and order while the wicked king and his sons thwarted every attempt.

Eventually all diplomacy was exhausted. Nothing was left but to go to war. And so the day came when the two opposing armies were massed on the battlefield eager to fight. But even yet, the rightful king wanted to be sure that fighting this war was right and necessary. His younger brother, Arjuna, the best among all warriors, rode out to take a final look at the kings and other warriors who were arrayed for battle.

The Dialogue Between Krishna and Arjuna

The great soul, Krishna himself, was the charioteer. Arjuna urged him to drive to the center of the battlefield so that he could see who had taken up arms against him and his brothers. What he saw was devastating—there with the opposing army stood his own grandfather, his teachers, cousins, nephews, and numberless other relatives and friends, ready to kill and be killed. His mind was flooded with despair. How could such a battle be anything but evil?

In his despondency, Arjuna turned to Krishna: "Oh Krishna, the best of the youth of both kingdoms stand here in this battlefield. Intoxicated by the opium of war, they have lost their senses. They think of nothing except killing. They are excited, they are blinded, they would rather die than retreat. Many of them will die—we will lose the better part of an entire generation of men.

"And that is only the beginning. When the war is over, the true catastrophe begins. Many in the older generation will die from grief; the younger generation will be bereft of guardians. The surviving mothers and sisters will become disoriented. People will suffer from the scarcity of food and clothing. Disease will thrive and there will be no one to treat the sick. Children will inherit only sadness and grief. Revenge and hatred will stalk the land.

"Don't you see, Krishna? This war will create a gap of three generations among us. It will shatter the civilization, culture, and knowledge which has flowed in an unbroken current from generation to generation for thousands of years. With the passage of time, the intensity of grief will subside and the normal human urges will return. But an entire generation of women will have no partners and so will suffer from adultery and other misconduct.

"Krishna, stop this war. I prefer to retire to the forest and live as monk rather than fight and gain a victory at such an unbearable cost—the loss of life, culture, civilization, natural resources, and ultimately, the wisdom of our ancestors."

"What possesses you, Arjuna? This is not the time to think of these things. The boundaries of these noble thoughts have already been crossed, and that is why we now stand on this battlefield. Even if you retire to the forest, these armies will clash. If, overwhelmed by these noble and peaceful thoughts, you do not fight, you will bear the entire responsibility for the destruction that will be wrought by your enemies. Even those that you lead are no longer in the mood for peace. These armies will spill each other's blood, no matter what you do. At least let righteousness triumph amidst this destruction.

"If you lead this army into battle, Arjuna, you might not get credit for the victory, but if you refuse to fight, you will certainly be blamed for failing to defend peace and justice. It's a bad bargain, but what can you do? That's what life is all about."

"You take life so lightly, Krishna! Can you really justify destruction and violence? Aren't we fighting for a piece of land and wealth? How can you value either of these more than life and peace? "

"Arjuna, you are walking backward. These are the thoughts that should come before armies gather, not in the midst of a battlefield. These questions are not flowing from the center of wisdom; they are only the manifestation of your attachment to your kinsmen, teachers, and friends.

"If your blood were not royal, it would not be your duty to lead a battle for kingdom and property. But your blood is royal, and you must preserve justice and order for the sake of your people. If you fail to do your duty, multitudes will suffer. Arjuna, in this light you are not a person, but a champion of essential human needs. You defend others by defending yourself. You must fight to protect others. This war is a means of avoiding a more severe and long-lasting injury. You must get up and fight."

"But Krishna, is nonviolence conditioned by time and place and circumstance? Is its application so limited? Tell me, oh my wise friend, when should one practice nonviolence and refuse to fight, even in self-defense? When should one defend oneself with arms? When should one surrender to the situation and when should one try to change it by any means possible—either peaceful or unpeaceful?"

"This is a profound question, Arjuna. There are two main ways of meeting any situation. All other ways come in between. These are the way of the tortoise and the way of the ocean. I will explain each of them to you. (See *The Gita*, chapter II, verses 58 & 70).

"Just as a tortoise, sensing a threat, withdraws into its shell and so remains safe, Arjuna, a human being should withdraw to safety when threatened. A tortoise never complains. Neither does it attack. Even if it receives a pounding, it does not fight. Yet it always wins because sooner or later the enemy retreats in frustration. With humans, the victory is even more complete, because a human enemy will be affected by the virtue of tolerance, forbearance, forgiveness, and passive resistance, and may even become a friend.

"The only difference between a human and a tortoise is that a tortoise is helpless and cannot choose to fight its enemy, whereas a human is not helpless and yet refrains from fighting. There is more power in voluntary inaction arising from the principle of nonviolence than in involuntary inaction arising from helplessness.

"Listen carefully, Arjuna. The way of the ocean is a higher path than the way of the tortoise. The ocean never rejects the waters of any river, whether polluted or clean, but allows all rivers to merge into it and, embracing them all, absorbs them as integral to itself. Such is the action of a human of the highest wisdom and greatest strength, who includes all and excludes none, loves all and hates none. People from all walks of life, people with different philosophies, abilities, and virtues are all embraced by the oceanic personality of such a one.

"Such people do not withdraw into protective shells when encountering a threat from 'enemies;' rather, they open the door of love and compassion and make themselves available to be loved or tortured. Even while being crucified, they utter no word of complaint. These are the people who transform society. Their inner strength surpasses the strength of millions. They are the torch bearers of the human race.

"You see, Arjuna, there are different paths for different people. The way of the ocean may better suit a renunciate or monk than the way of the tortoise. But the way of the tortoise is more suitable for one who has yet to transcend the confines of family, caste, and community and has yet to unfold the full breadth of inner strength and understanding. Each person must examine his or her own knowledge, understanding, inner strength, tolerance, forbearance, forgiveness, and compassion, to discover how to best to apply the principle of nonviolence. Ultimately, Arjuna, the only competent guide is one's own conscience, as long as it is not contradicted by common sense and the higher welfare of others."

"But Krishna, it doesn't answer the question of **when**

to surrender to the situation and when to try and change it."

"It is simple, Arjuna. Surrender to the situation if your personal life alone is affected. But take action if the lives of others are involved. If such a situation demands the use of force, use force."

"Yes, Krishna, but how do you justify the violence that attends the use of force?"

"Because you are a great man and you hold no animosity toward anyone, Arjuna, you must adhere to the way of the ocean. This is your personal path for private spiritual unfoldment. But you are more than a private person; you are also a public person entrusted with the welfare of the multitude. Personally you have no enemies because you are not contaminated by feelings of animosity. But the enemy of society, the enemy of the multitude, is absolutely your enemy. For the sake of humanity, this enemy must be vanquished.

"For your personal spiritual unfoldment, follow the path of the ocean, which is the path of the sages. But for the sake of humanity, follow the path of the noble warrior. By creating a balance between these two paths, you incur no sin in killing. Such action is called 'the action of an inactive person.'

"Fighting in a war while deep down practicing the principle of nonviolence is like rowing two boats at once. Only a master can row two boats and still reach the other shore safely. Such a task demands perfect balancebetween emotional reaction and rational decision. And you are the only one who can judge if you are successfully rowing two boats or if you are a hypocrite."

"Still, Krishna, this war, led by me and supported by a man of supreme wisdom like you, sets a dreadful example for future generations. My internal states—my thoughts, emotions, and beliefs—cannot be so easily transmitted to others. How can they discern them? People know me only through the example of my deeds. Some will take this example, and without understanding the subtleties of my internal states, will use it to justify committing violent deeds for their own convenience."

"Arjuna, humans have the intelligence to know that which they wish to know. If they wish to blind themselves, they can contradict the principles taught by their elders, misinterpret the clearest precepts, or twist the wisest teachings out of context. People have done this before now and they will do it again. These subtle principles are for those who have the courage to be honest with themselves and are willing to listen and understand.

"Therefore, Arjuna, do not take it amiss that your example will sometimes be exploited by the ignorant for their own selfish ends. No doubt you will be subject to harsh judgements, but that must not stop you from doing your duty. Defending righteousness and restoring law and order is your present duty.

"Don't degrade yourself to the point of impotence with these endless arguments, Arjuna. It's not like you.

Rise above this momentary weakness of your mind and heart. Get up like a warrior. Defend those who look to you for protection."

The Way Out

This dialogue between two learned heroes illustrates the complexity of deciding when to take up arms and defend righteousness at the cost of carnage and destruction. Viewed from one perspective, *The Bhagavad Gita* sets out to solve the riddle of war and ends up wrapping it in an enigma instead.

The text presents social, ethical, philosophical, and metaphysical reasons for fighting this particular war. These are thorny issues and, wise man that he is, Krishna skirts direct answers, discoursing instead on spiritual matters. Several times during the dialogue, Arjuna reminds his mentor of the practical issues at hand and asks for an unequivocal explanation of how it can be right for him to participate in a massacre that will destroy his kin, his race, and his country. But Krishna always reverts to metaphysical arguments—military council becomes spiritual instruction. This is because Krishna knows that spiritual knowledge is the only way through this morass; thus he continually directs the dialogue to the plane above the material.

Krishna urges Arjuna to fight, but will not do so

himself. Although he insists that this war is necessary, Krishna does not take up arms. He vows to stand with the forces of righteousness, yet he will not fight for them. He offers his presence, not his participation. The message implicit in this incongruity is that although human affairs may become so convoluted that war is inevitable, fighting will never eradicate the causes of war.

There are the times when matters become so tangled that war is unavoidable, even though it will not bring any permanent resolution. When a society is crumbling, laws are inhumane, people are suffering, and the only way to correct the situation is to overthrow the laws and the lawmakers, fighting may become a duty. That is a matter for each individual to decide. But even so, winning the war is only part of the mission. After the victory, it is crucial to find a way to restore harmony and justice. And this brings us back to the question of why human affairs become so convoluted in the first place.

The war in the *Gita* was instigated by possessiveness, as are most wars. As long as possessiveness abounds, war will recur. Excessive materialism is a dark crevice in the human heart where the light of spirituality has not yet penetrated. In this realm of darkness, we blindly steal what belongs to our neighbors, occupy each other's land, claim the fruits of others' labor, and attempt to satisfy our egos by dominating others and imposing our values on them. Until this darkness is banished, we will continue bruising ourselves and brutalizing others.

Just as we are blinded by materialism, our vision is obscured by our obsession with the current war, or the one just passed, or the one that is shaping itself. In our ignorance, we tell ourselves that when this particular war is over, justice will prevail, oppression will vanish, and life will be rosy. This is pure fantasy. The cause of war is spiritual blindness, and such a cause can never be removed at gunpoint. And that is why, even in the middle of the battlefield, Krishna imparts spiritual wisdom to Arjuna. He knows that if peace is to be more than an interval between two wars, the survivors must attain spiritual wisdom.

Once war begins, it is too late to debate whether or not it was inevitable. It is also useless to argue about who is right and who is wrong, because once the battle is joined, the combatants quickly lose all sense of fairness. Self-righteousness balloons on both sides, the justifications become more far fetched, and nothing matters anymore except winning. None of this is constructive. The problem of war is too complex for intellectual hypotheses, reasons, and justifications, as the following story illustrates:

> While walking through the forest, Buddha happened on a man who had just been shot with an arrow. The victim was grasping the arrow with both hands and gasping in pain. When Buddha knelt beside him, the wounded man unleashed a barrage of questions, "Who shot this arrow? Who is the

arrowmaker? What is the arrowhead made of? Which direction did the arrow come from? Why was I shot? When I find the answers to these questions, I will wipe those responsible from the face of this earth." With a loving look, Buddha replied, "First pull this arrow out. Staunch the bleeding. Put some medicine on the wound. Heal yourself. Then make your inquiries."

Spiritual wisdom is the only way we can heal ourselves. But the healing must be done skillfully. We must not mistake a particular set of religious practices for spiritual wisdom and busy ourselves with imposing them on others. To do so will reinfect the wound.

To cleanse and heal ourselves, we must apply only universal principles of spirituality—those which have the fewest religious overtones. Practices involving the purification of mind and heart and acceptance of others as our own brothers and sisters alone are helpful. In Buddhist and yogic literature, contemplating these principles is called *Brahma vihara*—living in God consciousness. The next chapter offers a practical approach to living in God consciousness.

Four

In the journey of life, the dust that rises and clouds the vision warns the traveller, "This is the road the crowd tramps, not the path the wise ones tread."

After the War:
Vanquishing Hatred and Revenge

O nce the fighting is over, people breathe a sigh of relief, clear the rubble, and pray that they will never have to face the pain and sorrow of war again. This is a sad and futile prayer. There has been no victory; the enemy has not been defeated. The real enemy, war itself, has simply gone underground with its weapons—anger, hatred, jealousy, greed, and revenge—intact. This deadly enemy camouflages itself with peace talks, political negotiations, territorial settlements, and war reparations. But because the spirit of war retains its commanders, soldiers, and weapons, these diplomatic maneuvers are ultimately ineffective. War always resurfaces.

Somewhere deep inside, we all know this, but we refuse to act on our knowledge. So far no one has devised a strategy for truly disarming the enemy and transforming the subtle agents of destruction into the generative forces of love, compassion, and mutual understanding. Instead, we concentrate on repairing the physical damage and get busy with building better weapons to defend ourselves in the future.

After any war—the periods following World War II and the Vietnam War in the United States, for example—people experiment with ways of channeling their energies in peaceful directions. But unfortunately, these experiments are rarely constructive or lasting. This is because we are attempting to create a new life with the same old mental patterns. This causes us to mistake sensual pleasure for happiness, material wealth for security, and chemically altered states for peace and relaxation.

During these periods in history, we end up satiated with sensory pleasures, smothered in material goods, stupefied by alcohol and other drugs, and thoroughly dissatisfied. So we are forced to try something else. Not knowing what we are searching for and thus having no idea where to look, our energy flows into the same old grooves—dominating others and trying to make ourselves feel powerful by forcing them to acknowledge our superiority. And so the cycle continues.

Once we recognize that the enemy is war itself and make a firm resolution to defeat this enemy once and for all, an enormous reservoir of energy becomes available. For example, the money and other resources that even a short war consumes can feed millions. The money required to build a B-52 bomber could also build a water treatment plant. The money spent in manufacturing gas masks could be used to educate children in one of the poorer countries. The time, energy, and ingenuity lavished on designing and testing a powerful new weapon could be used to develop an efficient irrigation system for a region stricken by drought. But do we really do such things? No—because we have not yet transformed our attitude toward ourselves and others. We have not yet really decided to live in peace and to let others live in peace.

Like war, peace begins at the individual level. We will stop fighting with other communities and nations when we stop fighting with our families and our neighbors. The animosity created when home is a battleground infects the community, engendering a collective atmosphere of animosity, which in turn infects the community of nations and makes the world a battleground.

People caught in personal and domestic battles either turn their anger inward and abuse themselves, or turn their anger outward and abuse their family members and quarrel with their neighbors. In either case, an atmosphere of hostility is generated which spreads in concentric circles. Jealousy, hatred, anger, possessiveness, and feelings of inferiority held at the individual level have the same effect as a stone dropped into a pond. The unrest ripples outward, disturbing the family, the community, the society, the nation, and finally, the community of nations.

It is not possible to quell the unrest in the larger world

until we have quieted our own restlessness. According to *The Yoga Sutra*, the most prominent text of yoga, there are four principles, which if cultivated and assimilated, will free our minds from the disturbances created by jealousy, hatred, anger, possessiveness, and feelings of inferiority. These four principles are friendship for those who are happy, compassion for those who are suffering, cheerfulness toward the virtuous, and indifference toward the so-called non-virtuous.

In the beginning, it may be difficult to discern the link between practicing these four principles and dissolving the feelings of anger, hatred, and revenge that fuel violence in the external world. But with time and practice, the link will become clear and our minds will become free of animosity and become established in God consciousness.

Living in God Consciousness: Four Practices

To live in God consciousness is to live without fear, anger, hatred, jealousy, and greed. These four principles have the power to give us this freedom. According to *The Yoga Sutra*, these principles can be practiced and assimilated either through contemplation or through meditation. Contemplation and meditation on these principles purify our minds and hearts. This purification will be accelerated by the courage to face our fears, the determination to transform our lives, the company of like-minded people, and the grace of God.

1. Friendship for Those Who Are Happy

Everyone wants to be happy. Thus, while trying to attain happiness, we constantly find ourselves surrounded by those striving for the same goal. We regard some of our fellow seekers as friends and others as competitors. Toward still others, we remain indifferent. But for the most part, our own insecurities and other weaknesses lead us to believe that the fewer candidates for happiness, the greater our own chances of achieving it. Therefore, at some subtle level, we want to get rid of everyone, even our friends, although life without friends is misery in itself. So, caught in the dilemma born of our own ignorance, we suffer from the pain we have created for ourselves.

There are endless permutations of this cycle. For example, when others succeed, even those we love, our own insecurity and feelings of inadequacy engender jealousy, and in subtle ways, our envy motivates us to attempt to destroy their happiness. Or, misguided by the tricks of our own minds, we sometimes delight in disturbing the happiness of others even at the cost of making ourselves unhappy.

This convoluted behavior is not confined to a particular

group, but is a widespread psychological disorder that cannot be cured by professionals. The only cure is self-transformation. What is required is an antidote for competitiveness and jealousy. That antidote is the attitude of friendliness for those who are happy and successful. Contemplation is one means of cultivating this attitude:

> **At least there is someone in the world who is happy. Let me learn to rejoice in the happiness of others. Let me walk on the path of happiness without elbowing others. Let me envision my happiness without clouding the happiness of others.**
>
> **Let me appreciate those who are already happy, and find ways to inspire those who are not. Let my happiness remain unaffected by others. Let me remember that the kingdom of happiness is infinite and eternal. If the whole world becomes happy, my happiness will grow rather than diminish.**

Examine your own circumstances and see how you are creating misery for yourself by envying the happiness of others. If you have neighbors who appear more fortunate than you, cultivate a friendly attitude toward them in your own mind as well as in your outward behavior. In this way, you begin to overcome your own feelings of inferiority, which are what torture you most.

Remember, this world is full of diverse beings, objects, thoughts, and feelings. Diversity is a law of nature. This diversity is characterized by an unequal distribution of intelligence, strength, wealth, and the inexplicable phenomenon of fate or providence. Therefore, expecting everyone to be equally happy is absurd, for this is not the design of nature. But neither is it the design of nature for humans to shoulder the task of accelerating the inequality among themselves and disturbing the natural peace and harmony of the world with jealousy and strife.

Another, more powerful means of developing an antidote for competitiveness and jealousy is to meditate on the concept of friendship. According to the sages, by meditating on the virtue of amity, one becomes the friend of all and the friend to all. Friendliness and animosity cannot coexist. The mere presence of a person who is fully established in the virtue of friendship neutralizes animosity in the hearts of others. In the presence of such a highly evolved person, one's internally held animosity washes away. This is called "the effect of company." The following story illustrates this point:

> **During the time of the Lord Buddha there lived a notorious cutthroat, the leader of a band of outlaws who roamed the land, terrorizing everyone in their path. The leader, the most ruthless of the lot, had sworn a solemn vow to behead 1,000 people with his own hands and make a garland of their fingers. He devoted himself to fulfilling his vow and, having severed 999 heads from the shoulders**

of the innocent, was impatiently seeking the ultimate victim.

While ranging through the thick forest, his men fell upon a lone traveler. Although the traveler offered no resistance, the brigands brought him before their leader at sword point, making no secret of the grisly fate that awaited him.

Eager to fulfill his vow, the chief drew his sword and growled, "First your fingers, then your head." Unperturbed, the captive, who happened to be the Lord Buddha, extended his hands saying, "If you have need of my fingers, my friend, take them and use them as you wish."

The cutthroat, staggered by this man who, moments from agony and death, remained gentle and undisturbed, began to quiver with terror. Buddha continued to gaze at him with love. The sword slipped from the chief's hand, and overwhelmed with remorse over all the blood he had spilled, the chief collapsed at the feet of the Enlightened One. Buddha touched his head, lifted him up, and in one loving embrace, banished every impulse to cruelty the man contained.

The next morning, the former cutthroat and all his men were ordained as monks. In Buddhist literature, this monk is known as Ananda, the most beloved disciple of Buddha.

Amity is an aspect of nonviolence. The clearest embodiment of this principle in modern times was Mahatma Gandhi, who taught his followers to "eliminate the animosity, not the enemy." Gandhi knew that the first step toward eliminating animosity was to perfect the principle of amity within himself. While out for a stroll one day, he happened on a group of children at play. At the sight of this thin, half-naked, altogether strange-looking man, the children took fright and fled. Gandhi loved children and called to them, hoping to allay their fears, but to no avail. This great soul paused for a moment, searched his mind and heart and concluded that a wisp of fear and animosity still lingered there, causing the children to flee. So he set himself to fasting and purifying his heart until the magnetism of his virtue of friendliness grew so powerful that it pulled children toward him.

When it is perfected, the virtue of amity is so powerful that all fear and animosity evaporate in its presence. But its real gift lies in the power it holds to banish all traces of jealousy and competitiveness from the thoughts, words, and actions of all who are earnestly striving to instill amity in their own hearts and minds.

2. Compassion for Those Who Are Suffering

Just as we pollute our minds and hearts with competitiveness and jealousy toward our happier and more successful neighbors, we also soil ourselves with feelings of superiority over those who are suffering. That same ego which is deflated by an encounter with someone who is happier than we are, swells at the sight of someone who is more miserable. Just as cultivating friendship for those who are happy dissolves competitiveness and jealousy, so cultivating compassion toward those who are in pain dissolves vanity and feelings of superiority.

Feelings of superiority are actually feelings of inferiority cloaked in vanity. As feelings of inferiority increase so does vanity, and sooner or later, this pernicious pair is bound to express itself in speech and action. Lack of concern for those who are less fortunate, scorning the unfortunate or feeling uncomfortable in their presence, and a general attitude of arrogance are the visible symptoms of feelings of inferiority.

As a result of these feelings, we build a thick wall between ourselves and those who are less fortunate. Because we fail to realize how damaging this wall is both to ourselves and to others, we continually add to it. Thus, balance is disturbed, differences increase, and the community fragments. The discontent that begins to smolder among those who are excluded inevitably blazes into hatred.

Honor and dignity are human birthrights. Blinded by ego, the happier and more fortunate among us fail to acknowledge this birthright in those who are weak and suffering, suppressing them with our arrogance or indifference. Failing to acknowledge another's pain is an act of violence. People suffer when their pain is ignored; those who are ignored or suppressed feel compelled to assert themselves in the name of honor and dignity. War is often the result.

The sages studied this problem and concluded that compassion for those who are suffering is the only remedy. Compassion is both subtle and profound. Although most people confuse compassion with sympathy, the resemblance between them is quite superficial. Sympathy is an emotional response to those in pain, and an emotional response presupposes identification. Compassion, on the other hand, is never accompanied by emotion and is a expression of pure, selfless love.

In sympathy, the internal state of the sympathizer is affected, but the compassionate person remains undisturbed. The sympathizer is reminded (either consciously or unconsciously) of similar experiences in his or her own life; thus the sympathetic response has past memories as its major cause. The person who is suffering is simply the stimulus for the sympathy.

Compassion is the fruit of wisdom and is completely unconditional; selfless service and pure love are the springs from which compassion flows. A person fully established in the principle of compassion expresses it effortlessly and is deeply concerned but unaffected. The compassionate person acts and moves on, with no interest in acknowledgement or reward.

In the process of learning to move from sympathy to compassion, the practitioner must be wary of acting on impulse and should take care not to become caught in the act of compassion itself, as the following vignette illustrates:

A young monk, a disciple of the Lord Buddha, was sitting on the bank of a flooded river. As he watched the water swirl by, he noticed a scorpion drowning. Thinking to save its life, he impulsively plucked it out of the water with his fingers. The scorpion promptly stung him. In surprise and pain, the monk dropped the scorpion back into the river, where it resumed drowning. Seeing this, the monk thought, "What else other than stinging can this poor fellow do? That's the way of scorpions."

Remembering the compassionate words of the Buddha, the inspired monk picked up the scorpion again, was stung again, and again dropped the scorpion in the river. This sequence was repeated over and over until every drop of the scorpion's venom had been injected into the monk. Only then was the determined man able to hold onto it long enough to drop it on the river bank. Half dead from the poison and the pain, the exhausted monk collapsed beside the spent scorpion.

As they lay there, an old monk happened along. The instant he saw the pair, he knew what had happened. He made a poultice for the youngster's swollen hand, and revived him. But as soon as the monk came to consciousness, the newcomer began slapping and scolding him. "Fool! Fool! Why invite such misery for yourself?"

The young monk was befuddled. "The scorpion was drowning. Haven't you heard our Lord's saying 'Compassion and love are the only wealth mankind possesses?' Selfless service is the law of life."

"Yes," the old monk replied, "It is true that you must perform your actions lovingly, compassionately, and selflessly, but most importantly, do it skillfully. This means, get a stick and use it to fish the scorpion out of the river. Once it's out, get away from it before it stings you."

We must learn to express our compassion through skillful service, selflessly rendered. Then we must walk away. Lingering compromises the virtue of selflessness, which is the essence of compassion. Suffering people have egos too and they need to retain their sense of dignity. On one hand, they need help, but they do not want to feel obligated or demeaned. Expect nothing, not even unspoken gratitude, from those to whom you render service. The ability to give is itself an act of grace, as the following story illustrates:

There once was a saintly Moslem poet named

Rahim. He was both very wealthy and very generous. Every morning he sat outside his door with an ample pile of grain, clothing, and money for anyone who might have need of these things. He offered these gifts with outstretched hands and downcast eyes— he never saw the people who received his bounty.

After this had been going on for years, another poet asked Rahim, "Why are you so shy and timid while giving these gifts? You seem almost to be ashamed."

Rahim replied, "All the objects in the world belong to God. It is God who gives those objects to the needy ones outside of my house every morning, using me as an instrument. I'm honored to be God's instrument. That's why I feel shy. But people mistake me for the true giver. That's why I feel ashamed."

Compassionate service helps to alleviate the pain of those who are suffering. But its greater value lies in purifying the minds and hearts of those who render it. The satisfaction and joy you derive from rendering selfless service to someone in need is immense and everlasting. However, there is one danger—feeding your ego by identifying yourself as a generous, compassionate person. This is destructive both to you and to those to whom you render service. Compassion is authentic only if your kind words and deeds are accompanied by subtle feelings of selflessness, lack of ego, and transcendence of the sense that "I am the doer."

All these factors can be held in the mind in one integral thought contained in the following contemplation:

> **All these people—those who are poor and suffering—are also children of God. By serving them, I am serving God. Let them express their gratitude only if it gives them pleasure. But let me remember that I don't deserve a syllable of thanks for my kind words or good deeds—these are simply my duty. I am thankful to those I serve because it is through them that I have been given the opportunity to serve God.**

Meditation on the principle of compassion is a means of erasing our own hatred, cruelty, and fear and replacing these traits with love, kindness, and a deeper understanding for others. Those who meditate on compassion rise above the primitive urge of self-preservation and thus, their reactions toward others are not motivated by fear. Such people spontaneously and effortlessly understand and forgive others. Those who are fully established in the principle of compassion know that the motivating factor behind most immoral, unethical, or non-virtuous actions is a lack of the basic necessities of life—either in the material, emotional, or spiritual realms. Therefore, no matter how many times a materially or spiritually impoverished person insults or harms one who is established in compassion, he or she continues to radiate selfless love.

3. Cheerfulness Toward Those Who Are Virtuous

Just as we want to be happy, we also want to be virtuous—or at least to think of ourselves as virtuous. Because of our habits of attachment, desire, ego, and vanity, most of us want others to recognize and applaud our virtue. Competitiveness and jealousy are as rampant in the realm of spirituality as they are in other spheres of life. Without examining our own minds and hearts, we criticize others, especially those who appear to be "closer to God" than we are. If for some reason, another's virtue is praised in public, most of us feel at least a twinge of jealousy. And when it comes to our religious and spiritual leaders, we are quick with our criticism and harsh in our judgements: "This guy is phoney." "What a hypocrite she is!" "Can you believe there are people foolish enough to believe in him and follow him?"

At the collective level, too, we compare our religious beliefs and spiritual practices with those of others, usually with the intention of finding fault and establishing the superiority of our path over theirs. In the external world, the damage caused by religious quarrels is unmistakable—history is replete with martyrs, crusades, pogroms, stonings, burnings, and every other imaginable form of violence committed in the name of God.

In the internal world, the damage caused by competing with others and judging their spiritual attainments is less visible, but no less devastating. Jealousy of fellow seekers and the habit of condemning and judging the path they have chosen pollutes our minds, separates us from others, and leads to violence. The antidote is to cultivate an attitude of cheerfulness and positive appreciation for those who appear to be more virtuous than we are.

The following is a contemplative practice for this particular principle:

> How delightful it is to see others on the path of virtue and righteousness. Any path, earnestly followed, will certainly lead a spiritual seeker to the highest truth. How grateful I am for those spiritually oriented people whose mere presence on this earth transforms the lives of others. They are the true servants of humanity. The virtues of love, compassion, and selflessness radiate from them. Let me appreciate them and learn from them.

One may also pray in the following manner:

> May I constantly remember, "God can verily be worshipped only by those who are more humble and tender than a blade of grass. God can verily be worshipped only by those who have more forbearance and tolerance than the tree that weathers fierce storms and scorching sun in perfect tranquility. God can verily be worshipped only by those who

constantly respect all without expecting the slightest respect from others.

Such a contemplative thought, which is a great virtue in itself, can flow spontaneously from our minds and hearts only if we ourselves are cheerful. Without inner cheerfulness, contemplating on the idea of cheerfulness toward others is artificial and becomes a rote mental exercise.

Cultivating Inner Cheerfulness

Cheerfulness is a spontaneous expression of a purified heart and a steady mind. A clear mind is naturally blessed with cheerfulness, and a cheerful person spontaneously loves all and hates none. A cheerful person is fulfilled within, and this cheerfulness overflows, affecting everyone who comes near. On the other hand, an impure mind teems with countless conflicts. Spiritually speaking, a person with such a mind is empty. One who is empty envies those who are fulfilled, and easily becomes angry and vengeful. Therefore, it is of utmost important to cultivate those divine qualities that purify the heart and steady the mind, thereby allowing cheerfulness to unfold spontaneously.

According to *The Bhagavad Gita*, the divine qualities are: fearlessness, steadfastness in knowledge, generosity, self-control, inclination toward studying the revealed scriptures, austerity, non-injury, truthfulness, self-sacrifice, tranquility, compassion, non-possessiveness, modesty, inner strength, forgiveness, fortitude, and absence of hatred and conceit. Unfolding these qualities transforms a person into a divine being.

There are numerous degrading qualities—among them egoism, ostentation, arrogance, conceit, anger, and rudeness—which are opposed to the divine qualities. These qualities entangle human beings in the web of insatiable desire, hypocrisy, arrogance, lust, anger, and strife and blind them to the knowledge that lust, anger, and greed are three gates that lead to perdition.

The *Gita* explains how to close these three gates and seal them permanently. This is done by systematically attenuating the degrading qualities and allowing the divine qualities to unfold in their stead. This scripture explains that every activity—physical, verbal, and mental—has three aspects: divine, intermediate, and demonic. By involving ourselves in activities that are intrinsically divine, we move closer to the Divine; the same is true of intermediate and demonic activities.

These three aspects permeate every sphere of action and have a profound influence on what we become. Thus, we can transform ourselves by becoming aware of how these aspects play out in our daily activities. Once we have attained this awareness, we can then begin to choose to drop the activities that have a demonic influence and engage in those that are divine.

This notion is somewhat alien to the habitual way most of us have come to regard the world. But a glance at these three aspects at play in a few of our activities will serve to clarify this concept and show how it can be used as a tool of transformation.

Food. Divine food is fresh, vibrant, easy to digest, lightly seasoned, cooked by someone who is serene, and earned without hurting others. Such food is pleasing to both our minds and our senses while it is being eaten and while it is being digested. Food which is nutritious but not fresh, and food which is mass-produced, or canned, or whose sole attractive features are appearance and taste, is intermediate food. Demonic food is old, smelly, devoid of nutrients, and painful to the sense of taste, smell, and sight. It is hard to digest and is injurious to our health.

Worship. Worship dedicated to God, selflessly, lovingly, and without demand or condition is divine worship. Worship dedicated to God or to other forces with the intention of securing a reward—such as power, fame, or material prosperity—is intermediate worship. Demonic worship is dedicated to ghosts and spirits.

Austerity. The highest austerity is performed with the single-minded will toward self-discipline, self-discovery, and self-purification. There is no thought of external recognition or reward because the practice is its own reward. The intermediate type of austerity is performed to demonstrate our virtue to others or to secure a higher post in a religious order. Demonic austerity is undertaken without joy or is imposed by external authority. Any practice of austerity which is a form of torture for the body or the mind is demonic.

Charity. A charitable act by a generous person who desires nothing in return, directed to the appropriate people at the perfect time, is the highest charity. Altruism and non-attachment to the result are the hallmarks of divine charity. Divine charity is a recognition of our oneness with others. But an act of charity performed with a motive, such as a desire to appear generous, is of the intermediate kind, even when it is enormously beneficial to the recipient. When an act of charity is coerced, or performed out of fear or under social or religious pressure, the act is painful and the memory of this painful act lingers in the mind. This kind of charity is demonic.

Discipline. There are three realms of discipline—physical, mental, and verbal. Serving others, cultivating a healthy body, and exercising control over the senses are examples of physical discipline. Speaking less, voicing only that which is true and sweet, and studying spiritual texts are verbal disciplines. Cultivating serenity of mind and mental silence, practicing inner control, and striving for purity of heart are forms of mental discipline.

These disciplines are divine when they are firmly grounded in self-knowledge and when we undertake them joyfully. If we undertake them without understanding why we are doing them or out of a sense of obligation, they are of an intermediate grade. And when these practices are forced on us by parents, teachers, religious institutions, or society, they become a form of torture, not a means of discipline. Thus, they lose their virtue and pull us toward the demonic.

The *Gita* contains similar descriptions of the effect of these three aspects on study, meditation, selfless service, and other spheres of action. The point is that by analyzing our physical, verbal, and mental activities in every area of life, we can transform ourselves and unfold our divine qualities. This is the work of a lifetime. It takes determination, courage, and the willingness to examine all of our habits and to consciously choose those that purify the mind and strengthen the will.

According to yoga, one who cultivates transparency of mind, clarity of thought, and firmness of will becomes light and cheerful. The more cheerful we are, the more difficult it is for painful thoughts to enter our minds. Painful thoughts create fear, insecurity, and delusion. And the less we have of these, the fewer negative feelings we will have for others. A mind unencumbered by negativity is open and spontaneous. Such a mind is clear and is quick to understand. The person possessing such a mind acknowledges and appreciates the virtues of others and is indifferent toward those who seem to be doing evil.

4. Indifference Toward the So-called Non-virtuous

We each have our own definition of "virtue." If someone is "non-virtuous" according to our definition, the judgmental part of our personality immediately comes forward and we label that person "bad." This colors our thought, speech, and action toward that person. We try to maintain a distance, either by withdrawing ourselves or by pushing them away from us. Or, we try to force them to change. Any of these actions sets the stage for violence.

Again, the only way to change this pattern is to change our own attitudes. We must realize that those whom we consider to be reprehensible or wicked are living according to their level of understanding. Trying to correct them by criticizing their way of life and values is counterproductive. According to yoga, if it is possible to model the higher values of love, compassion, selflessness, and non-possessiveness for the "non-virtuous," then that should be done. Often a glimpse of the higher virtues is enough to cause a person to reevaluate his or her behavior and to find a way to begin the process of self-transformation.

If we have not acquired the skill of leading such a person gently in the direction of self-transformation, the only other option is to cultivate an attitude of indifference—not for the doer but for the deeds. Developing an attitude of indifference toward those who we believe to be non-virtuous damages our sensitivity to others and destroys our capacity for forgiveness, kindness, and self-less love. By cultivating indifference toward the deeds themselves, we remain free of hostility while sending forth the positive energy of love and friendliness to the so-called non-virtuous.

This attitude of indifference is an act of nonviolence. In developing this attitude, we remain free of animosity for so-called non-virtuous people. We allow them their rightful place, and by refusing to associate the person with the deed, we avoid disturbing ourselves by becoming smug and punitive. By overlooking the lapses of others, we prevent the self-righteousness and discord that leads to violence and war.

The following contemplation is helpful in cultivating this attitude:

> **Let me not heed the actions of those who seem to be wicked or less righteous than me and those like me. Who am I to judge others? How often have I made the mistakes and done that which is not to be done?**
>
> **Even the most virtuous among us occasionally becomes involved in unworthy deeds or dishonorable behavior. Such things are common to human beings. Let me restrain my mind from dwelling on the apparent frailties of others. My goal is to remain tranquil and loving in the face of all actions.**

The End of War

Practicing these four principles will purify the mind and heart. Once we have developed friendship for those who are happy, compassion for those who are unhappy, cheerfulness toward those who are virtuous, and indifference to non-virtuous acts, we will no longer pose a threat to others and they will be neither defensive nor self-protective in our presence.

Pure love, compassion, selflessness, and self-acceptance radiate from us when we have purified our hearts. Because similar attracts similar, our presence will elicit these same qualities from others. And so love, compassion, cheerfulness, selflessness, and self-acceptance will begin to spread, radiating from the individual and infecting the community, the society, and finally the world. War will no longer be possible—there will be nothing left to fight about.

Imagine what a transformation will be wrought in the world when we have transformed ourselves. These four principles are so simple, yet so powerful. When we make them part of ourselves, we'll see only God when we look at others. We will become so open to those around us that we will become their souls and they ours. This is the state called "enlightenment."

According to the scriptures, enlightenment is not something that one achieves from the outside, but a spontaneous expression of the soul which unfolds when impurities are removed. Those who are enlightened may appear to live in the world and to walk among us, but in truth, they are living in God and walking in the kingdom of God. Because they are living in God, love is the only means they have of sharing their inner wealth.

Let us enlighten ourselves. Let us imbue ourselves with these four virtues and join the company of those whose wisdom is unsurpassed. Again and again the scriptures say that compassion and wisdom go hand in hand. The more compassion we have, the more wisdom we gain; perfection in wisdom is the ground for perfection in compassion. Perfection in compassion is the heart of nonviolence. We can achieve our genuine state of humanness by becoming wise, compassionate, loving, and nonviolent. And only when we become fully human will we truly understand what the scriptures mean when they say, "God created humans in His own image."

Peace, Peace, Peace.

Five

For the benefit of the soul, nature opens the Book of Life,
and turns the pages while we learn. Blessed are
those who read with attention and learn
the rhymes of eternity, silently singing the poem
of ecstasy to the Lord of Life.

Prayers for Peace

Universal Prayer

L ead me from the unreal to the real.
Lead me from darkness to light.
Lead me from mortality to immortality.
Peace, Peace, Peace.

Upanishads

Surrender

O h great, shining beings,
Through our ears may we hear
Only uplifting and auspicious words.
Through our eyes, may we see
Only that which is auspicious and
    beautiful.
Through our body and senses,
May we perform our actions
Fully dedicated to the Lord of Life.

With all our limbs intact,
And with our healthy bodies,
May we perform only those actions
Which support the functions of nature's
    forces,
And please the Supreme Lord.
Thus, by performing our actions lovingly
    and selflessly,
May we live one hundred years.

The Rig Veda

The Human Family

May we meet in harmony.
Transcending differences,
May we talk in harmony.
May we share what we know.
May we respect what we feel.
By following the path of the Sages,
May we find our rightful place,
And share the wealth granted us.

The Rig Veda

May there be harmony in our minds.
May there be harmony in our hearts.
May our perceptions be clear and
    peaceful.
May we be an ornament to mankind.

The Rig Veda

Thou shalt love the Lord thy God with all thy heart, and with all thy soul, and with all thy mind.

This is the first and great commandment. And the second is like unto it, Thou shalt love thy neighbor as thyself.

The New Testament
Matthew 22: 37-39

This we know: the earth does not belong to man, man belongs to the earth. All things are connected like the blood that unites us all. Man did not weave the web of life, he is merely a strand in it. Whatever he does to the web, he does to himself. As we are part of the land, you too are part of the land. This earth is precious to us. It is also precious to you. One thing we know. There is only one God. No man, be he Red Man or White Man, can be apart. We *are* brothers after all.

Chief Seattle
Letter to the US Government

Love

I t is a law that one cannot live without doing his duties, but it is also true that duties make the doer a slave. If the duties are performed skillfully and selflessly, then the duties do not bind the doer. All actions and duties performed with love become means in the path of liberation. Performing one's duty is very important, but more important is love, without which duty creates bondage. Fortunate is he who serves others selflessly and learns to cross the mire of delusion.

Swami Rama
Living with the Himalayan Masters

H e that loveth not, knoweth not God; for God is love.

The New Testament
John 4: 8

Divine Protection

Protect us together.
Nourish us together.
Make us prosperous and vibrant.
May the knowledge of the sages
Enlighten our lives.
May we never hate anyone.
Peace, Peace, Peace.

The Upanishads

Hatred stirreth up strifes: but love covereth
all sins.

The Old Testament
Proverbs 10:12

F orming a circle, gather together and place
thy bread in the center and share. You will
be granted the boon of living in a Godly circle
and God will share his love with you all.

From Islamic Scriptures

L et my plant bring forth Thy flowers.
Let my fruits produce Thy seed.
Let my heart become Thy lute, Beloved,
And my body Thy flute of reed.

Hazrat Inayat Khan
Sufi Order

Enemies

Ye have heard that it hath been said, Thou shalt love thy neighbor and hate thine enemy. But I say unto you, Love your enemies, bless them that curse you, do good to them that hate you, and pray for them which despitefully use you, and persecute you.

The New Testament
Matthew 5:43-44

Non–attachment

T he world manifests from God, exists in God, and is governed by God. Objects of the world are given to you, oh children of God, as gifts from the Source beyond. Enjoy the objects with full awareness that you are not the owner; never become attached to them. In any given circumstance, do not covet another's share.

Isha Upanishad

L ay not up for yourselves treasures upon earth, where moth and rust doth corrupt, and where thieves break through and steal: But lay up for yourselves treasures in heaven, where neither moth nor rust doth corrupt, and where thieves do not break through nor steal; For where your treasure is, there will be your heart also.

The New Testament
Matthew 6: 19-21

T hrough anticipation, one entertains an idea which in turn grows into attachment. From attachment there arises desire. From desire comes anger; from anger comes delusion; from delusion, loss of memory; from loss of memory, loss of discrimination. When discrimination is lost, a human being is doomed.

The Bhagavad Gita 2:62-63

Duty

Regarding pleasure and pain, gain and loss, victory and defeat as equal, fight the battle of life. In doing so, you will never incur sin.

The Bhagavad Gita, 2:38

Only the performance of your duty is your right, not the fruits of your actions. Neither let your actions be motivated by their intended fruits nor become attached to inaction.

The Bhagavad Gita, 2:47

Mind is bound by the law of karma.
And mind is released from the law of karma.
Mind's bondage binds man.
When mind is released he attains Nirvana.

Sayings of Saraha
From Buddhist Scriptures

Peace

May our secret acts nourish the common good.
May we meet in peace and harmony.
May our resolve be strong and thoughtful.
May our talks lead to protection and peace.
Through our actions, may we invoke peace
and honor the Truth that resides in all.

The Rig Veda

Blessed are the merciful: for they shall obtain
mercy. Blessed are the pure in heart: for they
shall see God. Blessed are the peacemakers:
for they shall be called the children of God.

The New Testament
Matthew 5:7-9

O h peacemaker, before trying to make peace throughout the world, first make peace within thyself.

Hazrat Inayat Khan
Sufi Order

A nd they shall beat their swords into plow-shares, and the spears into pruninghooks: nation shall not lift up sword against nation, neither shall they learn war any more.

The Old Testament
Isaiah 2:4

Cheerfulness

 t last, said the Master, "No matter where you live, live cheerfully. This is the mantra. Be cheerful at all times, even if you are behind bars. Anywhere you live, even if you have to go to a hellish place, create heaven there. Remember, my boy, cheerfulness is of your own making. It only requires human effort. You have to create cheerfulness for yourself. Remember this mantra of mine."

Swami Rama
Living with the Himalayan Masters

Fear and Danger

Fear gives birth to insecurity which creates imbalance in the mind, and this influences one's behavior. A phobia can control human life and finally lead one to the insane asylum. If a fear is examined, it will usually be found to be based on imagination, but that imagination can create a kind of reality. It is true that fear invites danger, and human beings then must protect themselves from that self-created danger. All of our dreams materialize sooner or later. Thus it is really fear that invites danger, though we usually think that danger brings on the fear.

Swami Rama
Living with the Himalayan Masters

Truth

T ruth is the ultimate goal of human life, and if it is practiced with mind, speech and action, the goal can be reached. Truth can be attained by practicing non-lying and by not doing those actions which are against one's own conscience. Conscience is the best of guides.

Swami Rama
Living with the Himalayan Masters

H e created the heaven and the earth with the Truth. Highly exalted be He above what they associate with Him.

The Koran
Surah 16B

ll, from biggest stars to the tiniest speck of dust, is pervaded by Truth. But the face of Truth is hidden by the golden disc of worldly charms and temptations. Oh Nourisher and Eternal Guide of my Life, lift this veil so that I can see the Truth in its full glory.

Isha Upanishad

Self-mastery

I t is important to make one's life creative and helpful, but before doing so, one should make contact with his own potentials deep within by disciplining himself and gaining control over his mind, speech and action... A person who has gained such self-mastery lives in the world and yet remains above it unaffected by worldly fetters and problems.

> *Swami Rama*
> *Living with the Himalayan Masters*

J ust as the tortoise withdraws its limbs, so when a human withdraws his senses from the sense objects, his wisdom becomes steady. When a man is free from ego and desire, attachment and aversion, when he entertains and hates none, his wisdom naturally becomes firm.

> *The Bhagavad Gita 2:58*

Purification

O ne who has neither purified his mind nor controlled his senses, and yet tries to enjoy worldly pleasures is like a bird that flies from a ship in the ocean but, not seeing the land, comes back in frustration.

From Buddhist Scriptures

W hile enjoying the objects of the world, a human being can keep the mind clean and pure only by attaining freedom from attachment and aversion, and thereby gaining self-mastery. Clarity of mind eliminates all pains and miseries. It is only in the purified mind-field that truth is revealed from the source beyond. An undisciplined person has neither right knowledge nor right thinking. How can a person who neither knows rightly nor thinks rightly ever be happy?

The Bhagavad Gita, 2:64-66

I ncrease your capacity. Purify yourself. Acquire that gentle strength within. God will come and say to you, 'I want to enter this living temple that you are.' Prepare yourself for that situation. Remove the impurities and you will find that he who wants to know reality is himself the source of reality.

Swami Rama
Living with the Himalayan Masters

S tudy your thoughts and you will know what your mind is made of. That study begins by having confidence in the words of your wise Master. That study is none other than the process of meditation. That clears your mind and removes confusion. Cleanse your mind by cleansing your thoughts. Only then will you understand the intent of the Master's words.

From Buddhist Scriptures
Saying of Saraha

The Journey of Life

I n the journey of life, nature provides this body as a chariot. The senses are the horses; mind, the reins; and the power of discrimination is the charioteer—the guiding force. In this chariot sits the soul. The soul completes the journey and reaches the goal if the chariot is strong, the horses are trained, and the charioteer knows how to drive on the right path. Listen, oh human beings, the loss of the chariot is not a major loss; the real loss is not reaching the goal before the chariot falls apart.

Katha Upanishad

Many in the world are fully deluded yet claim and pose to be learned and wise. How sad is the fate of those who are blind and led by the blind. Wake up, oh child of light. Get up determined to walk and find those who are fully awake. Gather knowledge from those who have already found it, but remember, you must summon the courage to walk the razor's edge.

Katha Upanishad

Light

Yet a little while is the light with you. Walk while ye have the light, lest darkness come upon you: for he that walketh in darkness knoweth not whither he goeth.

While ye have light , believe in the light, that ye may be the children of light.

The New Testament
John 12:35-36

Ye are the light of the world. A city that is set upon a hill cannot be hid.

Neither do men light a candle, and put it under a bushel, but on a candlestick; and it giveth light unto all that are in the house.

Let your light so shine before men, that they may see your good works, and glorify your Father which is in heaven.

The New Testament
Matthew 5:14-16

Epilogue

Be ye therefore perfect, even as your Father which is in heaven is perfect.

The New Testament
Matthew 5:48

Judge not that ye be not judged. . . And why beholdest thou the mote that is in thy brother's eye, but considerest not the beam that is in thine own eye?

The New Testament
Matthew 7:1,3

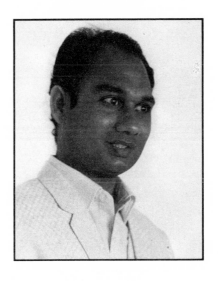

Pandit Rajmani Tigunait, Ph.D., a disciple of Sri Swami Rama of the Himalayas, is Spiritual Director of the Himalayan International Institute. In addition to his spiritual training, he has studied all branches of Indian philosophy and ancient scriptures, including the Vedas and the Upanishads. He received his higher education from the universities at Benares and Allahabad in India, and from the University of Pennsylvania. Pandit Tigunait serves on the faculty of the graduate Program in Holistic Studies at the Himalayan Institute. He is the author of *Seven Systems of Indian Philosophy.*

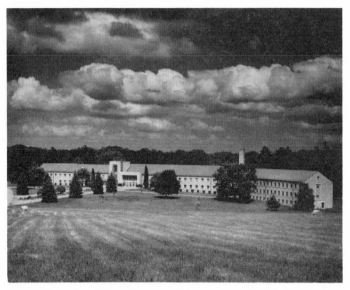
The main building of the national headquarters, Honesdale, Pa.

The Himalayan Institute

The Himalayan International Institute of Yoga Science and Philosophy of the U.S.A. is a nonprofit organization devoted to the scientific and spiritual progress of modern humanity. Founded in 1971 by Sri Swami Rama, the Institute combines Western and Eastern teachings and techniques to develop educational, therapeutic, and research programs for serving people in today's world. The goals of the Institute are to teach meditational techniques for the growth of individuals and their society, to make known the harmonious view of world religions and philosophies, and to undertake scientific research for the benefit of humankind.

This challenging task is met by people of all ages, all walks of life, and all faiths who attend and participate in the Institute courses and seminars. These programs, which are given on a continuing basis, are designed in order that one may discover for oneself how to live more creatively. In the words of Swami Rama, "By being aware of one's own potential and abilities, one can become a perfect citizen, help the nation, and serve humanity."

The Institute has branch centers and affiliates throughout the United States. The 422-acre campus of the national headquarters, located in the Pocono Mountains of northeastern Pennsylvania, serves as the coordination center for all the Institute activities, which include a wide variety of innovative programs in education, research, and therapy, combining Eastern and Western approaches to self-awareness and self-directed change.

SEMINARS, LECTURES, WORKSHOPS, and CLASSES are available throughout the year, providing intensive training and experience in such topics as Superconscious Meditation, hatha yoga, philosophy, psychology, and various aspects of personal growth and holistic health. The *Himalayan Institute Quarterly Guide to Classes and Other Offerings* is sent free of charge to everyone on the Institute's mailing list.

The RESIDENTIAL and SELF-TRANSFORMATION PROGRAMS provide training in the basic yoga disciplines—diet, ethical behavior, hatha yoga, and meditation. Students are also given guidance in a philosophy of living in a community environment.

The PROGRAM IN HOLISTIC STUDIES offers a unique and systematic synthesis of Western empirical sources and Eastern introspective science. Graduate-level studies may be pursued through cross - registration with several accredited colleges and universities.

The five-day STRESS MANAGEMENT/PHYSICAL FITNESS PROGRAM offers practical and individualized training that can be used to control the stress response. This includes biofeedback, relaxation skills, exercise, diet, breathing techniques, and meditation.

A yearly INTERNATIONAL CONGRESS, sponsored by the Institute, is devoted to the scientific and spiritual progress of modern humanity. Through lectures, workshops, seminars, and practical demonstrations, it provides a forum for professionals and lay people to share their knowledge and research.

The ELEANOR N. DANA RESEARCH LABORATORY is the psychophysiological laboratory of the Institute, specializing in research on breathing, meditation, holistic therapies, and stress and relaxed states. The laboratory is fully equipped for exercise stress testing and psychophysiological measurements, including brain waves, patterns of respiration, heart rate changes, and muscle tension. The staff investigates Eastern teachings through studies based on Western experimental techniques.